The Clinical Educator – R

For Churchill Livingstone:

Editorial director (Nursing and Allied Health): Mary Law
Project manager: Valerie Burgess
Project editor: Dinah Thom
Copy editor: Adam Campbell
Project controller: Derek Robertson
Design direction: Judith Wright
Sales promotion executive: Maria O'Connor

The Clinical Educator – Role Development

A self–directed learning text

Ann P Moore PhD MCSP DipTP Cert Ed MACP
Deputy Head, Department of Occupational Therapy and Physiotherapy,
University of Brighton, Eastbourne

Ros W Hilton MSc DPHE MCSP DipTP
Post-Graduate Course Co-ordinator and Senior Lecturer, Physiotherapy Group,
Biomedical Sciences Division, King's College, London

D Jane Morris MCSP
Clinical Educator Tutor, Physiotherapy Group,
Biomedical Sciences Division, King's College, London

Lynne K Caladine MSc MCSP DipTP
Course Leader (Bsc (Hons) in Physiotherapy) and Senior Lecturer, Department of
Occupational Therapy and Physiotherapy, University of Brighton, Eastbourne

Helen R Bristow MSc MCSP
Formerly Human Resources Development Manager (Physiotherapy) and
Clinical Placements Liaison Officer, South East Thames Regional Health Authority

Foreword by
Alan Walker MA
Director of Education, Chartered Society of Physiotherapy, London

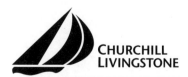
**CHURCHILL
LIVINGSTONE**

NEW YORK EDINBURGH LONDON MADRID MELBOURNE SAN FRANCISCO AND TOKYO 1997

CHURCHILL LIVINGSTONE
Medical Division of Pearson Professional Limited

Distributed in the United States of America by Churchill
Livingstone, 650 Avenue of the Americas, New York, N.Y.
10011, and by associated companies, branches and
representatives throughout the world.

First published 1997

ISBN 0 443 05300 6

British Library Cataloguing in Publication Data
A catalogue record for this book is available from the British
Library.

Library of Congress Cataloging in Publication Data
A catalog record for this book is available from the Library
of Congress.

The
publisher's
policy is to use
**paper manufactured
from sustainable forests**

Produced through Longman Malaysia, PP

Contents

Foreword

Physiotherapy is a practical profession where the term 'hands-on' has a literal meaning. It is therefore not surprising that physiotherapy education should be firmly rooted in practice. No less then 1000 hours of qualifying programmes must be devoted to clinical education, and it is impossible for any student to qualify as a chartered physiotherapist unless all clinical placements have been successfully completed.

This emphasis on practical experience has served to maintain and enhance the standards of care provided by physiotherapists. It may also, however, result in limitations being placed on the learning process itself. The very immediacy of physiotherapy education, with its culture of clinical skills and role models, has meant that the enormous potential of open learning has rarely been exploited. Now, if ever, is the time for these traditional attitudes to be challenged. The health care industry, as with all modern life, stands on an exponential curve of advancing technology which will increasingly alter the ways in which people communicate and learn. Physiotherapy education must adapt to these changing factors, without forgetting that health care is forged on human contact and empathy.

Nowhere in physiotherapy education is human contact more vital than in a student's clinical experience. It is therefore encouraging that this topic should form the focus of an open learning pack, developed by the University of Brighton and King's College London, which aims to promote the human issue of role development for clinical educators by the technical means of open learning. The pack represents a valuable means of promoting high standards of clinical education, while also providing accessible educational opportunities for practising physiotherapists and other health care professionals.

I hope that you, as clinical educators, enjoy using this pack, and that it helps to extend your role and practice.

London, 1996   AW

Preface

The future of any healthcare profession is largely dependent on the quality of the education it provides for its future generation. Clinical education forms an essential part of this process and provides the opportunity to consolidate theory with practice, to enhance practical skills and to prepare the student for professional life. Thus, there is a consensus amongst the various health professionals that clinical education is a crucial course component. In recognising this fact, we must strive to ensure that those senior practitioners who are responsible for clinical education are encouraged continually to develop in their role as clinical educators.

We, the authors, are five chartered physiotherapists who have worked collaboratively over the last five years to develop physiotherapy clinical education on behalf of the students and clinicians involved with two undergraduate courses and for a number of postgraduate students on a range of courses.

It is our experience that time and financial constraints on clinical physiotherapists reduce the number of educational courses that they attend. Physiotherapists will frequently choose to attend a course that updates or develops their specialist clinical, rather than educative, skills. It is for these reasons that this text has evolved as a learning package. Through reflection, discussion, reading, and work-based and theoretical assignments, you will be encouraged and supported to develop and extend your role as a clinical educator.

The package is intended to address the concept of education in the clinical environment in its broadest sense and therefore to meet the needs of clinicians who are involved in the education of learners, other healthcare professionals, junior staff, patients, clients, carers or members of the public. We appreciate that this intention, and the content and skills development addressed in this package, will be of interest to members of other healthcare professions who are involved in clinical education. However, our primary aim is to encourage and facilitate the development of this role in physiotherapists who are currently in practice as well as those who are returning to clinical practice. Consequently, most of the activities focus on physiotherapy related issues and the main emphasis will be on working with learner physiotherapists and junior staff. Readers who are members of other healthcare disciplines should find the content applicable to their own practice settings but may care to refer to their own professional literature for specific references and other useful material.

This package could supplement any personal development programmes which higher education institutions offer in support of clinical education development.

Brighton and London, 1996

APM,
RWH,
DJM,
LC,
HRB

Introduction

Welcome to this learning package, which has been developed in open-learning format primarily for physiotherapists who are engaged in the education of others in clinical workplace settings and who wish to develop their skills as clinical educators.

The aims of this package are:

- to provide you with a clear understanding of the term 'clinical educator'
- to enhance your contribution to the education of others in both clinical and other workplace settings
- to develop your understanding of the role of the clinical educator
- to enable you to consider your role as an educator in today's healthcare climate
- to enable you to create a favourable learning environment
- to enhance your understanding of how adults may approach learning, with direct reference to learning theories
- to enable you to assess and evaluate learning
- to help you to understand the purpose and context of clinical education
- to help you to plan learning experiences.

It is fundamental to good practice that the learner identifies what they hope to achieve before embarking on any learning experience. So, to begin with, it would be useful for you to think about what you hope to achieve by using this package.

ACTIVITY I.1

Write down your personal reasons for working through this package and what you hope to achieve by the end of it. At the beginning and end of each section you may find it useful to review this list, as it should help you plan your work and consider whether your objectives have been achieved.

How to use this package

There are two parts to this package, the self-directed learning text and the Reader. They are designed so that you can study independently or in a small group at whatever pace you wish. However you decide to study, you should try, wherever possible, to apply the concepts addressed in the text to your own particular working environment and also to reflect on your own, and others', practice in terms of clinical education. Wherever possible, investigate the educational practices and philosophies used by other health professions. If possible, and appropriate, study with a multidisciplinary group so that you can gain from the clinical education experiences of other professions.

Structure of the learning package

The text in each section includes an introduction, an aim and a set of learning objectives which identify goals that you should have achieved by the end of the section.

Activities are interspersed throughout the text to help you successfully achieve the learning objectives.

These include:

- short written assignments
- short interviews with learners / peers
- developing flow charts to show relationships between ideas / concepts
- planning a learning experience
- reflection on ideas put forward on new concepts
- summarising / reflecting on your own skills, attitudes, experience, knowledge and those of your learners or peers.

In addition, and where appropriate, reflective self-assessment exercises are inserted into the text to help you to evaluate whether you are learning effectively and to assess the quality of your own learning. Keep all of your written responses to the Activities as they will be useful as you work through Section 11. Some Activities have time allocations to give you an idea of the breadth / depth of study required. These times are meant to be indicative rather than prescriptive.

Outlines of the sections
There are twelve sections to this study guide:

Section 1 – An overview of clinical education
Explores the concept of clinical education within the present changing climate of health and education provision.

Section 2 – The role of the clinical educator
Analyses the role of the clinical educator in terms of the knowledge, skills and attitudes necessary to be an effective educator.

Section 3 – Identifying the learner and educator and their interactions
Identifies who the learners are in the clinical education setting and explores some of the characteristics of educators and learners, and the relationships which may occur between them.

Section 4 – Learning theories
Introduces theories that relate specifically to adult and professional learning.

Section 5 – Factors influencing learning
Considers the major internal and external factors influencing learning, such as the environment, and physiological and psycho-social dimensions.

Section 6 – The learning environment
Helps you to create a learning environment which is suitable for the needs of your learners.

Section 7 – Facilitating learning
Helps you to plan the learning experience and enables you to decide the most suitable approaches to learning in the workplace, including reference to learning contracts.

Section 8 – Assessment
Addresses issues related to the assessment of learning in the clinical workplace and includes the what, who, why and how of assessment.

Section 9 – Evaluating learning
Explores ways in which you can evaluate whether learning has taken place and the quality of that learning. Enables you to formulate action plans relating to the evaluation process and outcomes of the learning experience.

Section 10 – The development and purpose of clinical education
Initiates deeper consideration of the purpose and development of clinical education and raises awareness of relevant professional developments.

Section 11 – The learning experience model in action
A series of consolidatory self-assessment exercises.

Section 12 – Further information
Provides contact addresses for information on opportunities for further study and gives a list of further reading to enable you to deepen your knowledge and interest in clinical education.

Appendix 1
Factors which influence learning as identified by learners

Appendix 2
An example of a clinical placement assessment form

Appendix 3
An example of a clinical placement evaluation form

Glossary
A glossary of key terms has been included to aid your study.

1 An overview of clinical education

Introduction

For many years the education of health professionals has involved a blend of college and workplace learning. In turn, many practitioners have gone on, by choice or through the demands of their own clinical post, to contribute to the education of learners in their clinical field. Within our changing world, this part of the educational process has also been evolving, in ways that may or may not be obvious to those involved.

Aim

In this opening section we will explore the concept of clinical education within the present, changing climate of health and education provision.

Objectives

When you have completed this section you should be able to:

1. Identify the key players in the clinical education setting.
2. Recognise the settings in which clinical education occurs.
3. Demonstrate an insight into the development of clinical education in light of the current changes in health and higher education.
4. See how you as an individual professional can contribute to the education process.

As each profession uses different terms for the various parts of the clinical education process, we first need to clarify those that will be used throughout this self-directed learning pack.

Clinical education

This is the essential and most wide-ranging element of healthcare professional courses which takes place in numerous and diverse settings and circumstances. It 'provides the focus for the integration of academic and practice based learning' in a work-based setting (The Chartered Society of Physiotherapy 1991).

Pre-registration education (and also much clinical post-registration education) for healthcare professionals involves a combination of college- and practice-based teaching. The latter is achieved through a series of work-based clinical placements, where the learner undertakes supervised learning and practice in a relevant service setting. During these placements, a practitioner is involved in educating and assessing the learner.

Clinical educator

The 'clinical educator' is an experienced work-based professional practitioner who accepts responsibility for a specific part of the clinical education process. Clinical educators are normally senior practitioners with a high level of clinical knowledge, and extensive skills and experience, in a specialist field. In addition, they may be responsible for the daily management of their clinical units and for personal caseloads. Their activities may involve the education of others, including junior staff, patients and carers.

Where the clinical educator is responsible for a learner on an undergraduate or postgraduate course, the responsibility for clinical education is shared with the educators from the learner's college base.

Learner

Generally, in this context, the 'learner' is an undergraduate, or a qualified member of a healthcare profession, who is undertaking a clinically based education programme. Every learner undergoes a series of work-based placements in a variety of service environments. The pattern, duration and range of clinical education experience will vary according to the design of the course and the availability of placements in specific clinical areas. However, the total profile should accurately reflect current clinical practice in the professional area, thereby helping to prepare the learner for independent work in the field. The overall programme is devised by the learner's course tutors in conjunction with the managers of the provider services that support the course.

In the case of undergraduate healthcare professionals, this programme will include placements in a range of relevant primary and secondary health and social care services, such as acute hospitals, local health centres, GP practices, the client's own home, residential homes, day centres, schools and centres of leisure and of employment. Wherever the setting, each placement has unique features which will impact on the planned learning process and on the achievement of the programme objectives. The significance of these factors will be addressed further in Section 6.

ACTIVITY 1.1

Please keep some notes of your thoughts on this activity so you can refer back to them later.

Spend about 10 minutes thinking about the above definitions and reflecting upon the following:

Recall the placement profile you had as a pre-registration learner, the type of services your placements were in and their duration.

If your placements varied significantly in length, consider the relative merits and disadvantages of the duration of each.

Does a typical placement profile of an undergraduate learner today resemble your own experience as a learner? If not, consider the range of factors which have been responsible for the changes.

If possible, discuss this last part with members of other healthcare professions with whom you now work. Are the factors the same for each profession?

Development of clinical education in healthcare professional education

Bond (1990) surveyed 10 healthcare professions for the Health and Care Professions Education Forum (H&C PEF; see description at the end of the section) and showed that the system used in the preparation of clinical educators is both complex and variable. The preparation normally occurs during unidisciplinary courses which vary from one profession to another in organisation, availability, duration and content. While the provision of clinical work-based placements has been a feature of health professional education for many years, very little research has been undertaken into exactly how one learns in work-based environments, and how educators should assist this learning process. You will find references to the relevant research at appropriate points throughout the package.

Historically, many pre-registration learner groups were regarded as the junior part of the professional workforce, learning by 'apprenticeship'. However, in recent years the majority of healthcare professions have moved to all graduate entry, and their preregistration courses have moved into the higher education sector. This change has been accompanied by the growing recognition that the clinical component is an essential element of the overall educational programme and that learners should in fact be supernumerary to the workforce. As a result, some clinical educators now participate in the planning, development and evaluation of the courses they are involved in, and individual clinical educators participate in the assessment of learners in the workplace.

Current issues influencing clinical education

In recent years, the organisation of both health and education provision has changed substantially. The short-term instability created as a result of these changes has inevitably had a significant impact on the provision of clinical education. From some perspectives, these changes have been detrimental. For example, a number of college-based clinical co-ordinators have reported securing inappropriate numbers of clinical placements for their learners. When such difficulties arise, clinical colleagues report fluctuations in their senior staff establishments as a constraint.

Health provision

As a result of the health service reforms which followed the NHS & Community Care Act (1990), total responsibility for the delivery of health services was split between health 'purchasers' and service 'providers'. The purchasers operate on a local basis and are legally required to ensure that the health needs of their local population are identified and catered for. This is done by purchasing the relevant services from a range of providers. In this way, a 'market economy' has been introduced into the health service in the UK. Market forces have therefore become a prevailing factor, and service costs, benefits and quality are now being scrutinised carefully. The 'activity' of clinical education inevitably comes under such scrutiny.

Education provision

Healthcare professional education was traditionally offered in National Health Service 'schools' which were allocated to, or associated with, local health districts. Professional educators were NHS employees whose sole remit was the preparation of learners for healthcare practice.

Courses were always demanding and, in the main, led to a professional qualification at diploma level.

Throughout the 1980s, several professional groups decided that it was desirable for learners entering their profession to do so with graduate status. For most groups this involved a move into the higher education sector. With this new arrangement, the input of educators from the professions could be complemented by the experience of academics from disciplines that influence healthcare professional practice.

Drawing upon a wide range of expertise, courses were developed with the aim of equipping learners for the current demanding and changing world of healthcare.

The process of awarding and validating degrees is controlled and administered by Universities. However, in most cases, courses for healthcare professionals are approved by both the host institution and the appropriate professional body so that a licence to practise is granted at the same time.

This new process has embraced learners and teachers, with educators from the professions now being required to fulfil responsibilities in teaching, management and research.

While ownership of the educational process now falls almost wholly within the education sector, the funding of this education and decisions concerning the future supply of trained personnel remain the responsibility of the health sector. Consequently, there is a potential for tension between the two sectors with respect to funding arrangements. This was recognised when the reforms were introduced, and in an endeavour to safeguard health professional training from the financial pressures on the health service, Working Paper 10 (NHS & Community Care Act 1990) was drawn up. The principle of Working Paper 10 was that healthcare professional workforce planning and education commissioning should be the responsibility of local health employers and be coordinated by regional health authorities (RHAs). So far, this has been achieved by RHAs in the following way. They conduct surveys of local manpower demand and then place contracts with appropriate higher education institutions for the desired number of qualifying learners. These numbers are, of course, subject to central monitoring and where necessary they are adjusted to suit.

However, at the time of writing, it is central policy that the existing RHAs' functions will be removed in 1996 and ongoing arrangements for their current non-statutory responsibilities, such as education and manpower planning, are not yet clear. Brook (1994) concludes that 'new policies in healthcare will inevitably influence . . . the educational process.' It is not yet clear how the process will actually be affected, but, as we have seen, some current policies are already making clinical education vulnerable. For example, in an effort to safeguard placements, the notion of educational institutions accrediting and contracting work-based placements is currently being discussed by professionals.

ACTIVITY 1.2

We suggest you read the following two articles in the Reader (pp 1& 3) before proceeding further with this pack. They will provide you with a comprehensive summary of recent relevant developments in physiotherapy education and the central policy changes which have affected it up until the demise of RHAs in 1996.

In the Walker article please note that the circumstances described are historical to that period (1991) and that the reference to the Society's new curriculum of study relates to the 1991 curriculum.

1. Walker A 1991 Clinical education – funding and standards. Physiotherapy 77 (11): 742–743
2. Brook N 1994 A sharp intake of breath: inspirations in education – some of the issues. Physiotherapy 80 (A): 20–23

Clinical education and the professional role

Upon the successful completion of an undergraduate healthcare course, learners receive an academic award and also become eligible for membership of the relevant professional body. Hence, one broad aim of their education is to produce competent and adaptable practising professionals, thereby securing the supply for the next generation.

Professionals may be described as members of an archetypal occupational group or 'clan' whose roles are predominantly maintained by unobtrusive cultural controls. The traditional professions of the Law, Medicine, Church and the Military have been joined over the last 150 years by many others, including a number of health and social care professions. However, all share a number of characteristics (Dawson 1992):

● commitment to a distinct body of knowledge
● specific and lengthy training
● restrictive entry
● prescribed code of ethics and standards of behaviour
● proclaimed concern for client groups
● peer group evaluation, control and promotion.

Thus, as a senior practitioner involved in workplace education, you are in a very powerful position to influence and guide learners towards professional competence and to affect both how much they learn and the quality of their learning. Emery (1984) shows that in the workplace setting the learner develops through 'learning by doing' and through being given the opportunity to recognise their experiential learning – i.e. having adequate time and support to analyse, reflect and evaluate their experience. The significance of your power in this respect cannot be underestimated. We will consider this further in Sections 2 and 6, and also at various other points throughout the pack.

ACTIVITY 1.3

Aim to spend about 15 minutes completing this activity.

Note down, in any style you wish, the specific characteristics of the physiotherapy profession, as identified by Dawson (1992, p. 32).

Consider how your current interaction with physiotherapy learners enables you to demonstrate good professional practice as a role model.

Professional rules of conduct and standards of good practice

As has already been implied, each healthcare professional body has its own remit, rules of professional conduct, disciplinary procedures and structure. Many professions have also recently developed standards as guidelines for good practice, in order to bring about the continued evaluation and promotion of their profession.

Clearly, when dealing with rules and guidelines such as these, it is likely that there will be local variations in how rigorously they are interpreted and also in how the standards are applied. Given that most learners will undertake their clinical education in a variety of service settings, they are likely to come across senior practitioners who will interpret the standards and rules differently. Initially, learners may be confused about what level of professional behaviour is required or expected of them. The development of the learners' professional competence is dependent upon the growth of their professional judgement. Acquiring this judgement is something they will find challenging, especially early on in their clinical careers.

ACTIVITY 1.4

Spend about 5 minutes on this activity.

Consider your own professional body (i.e. The Chartered Society of Physiotherapy). In what ways do you think it contributes to the education process of your profession?

ACTIVITY 1.5

Spend about 15 minutes on this activity.

Reflect upon your own clinical experiences as a learner and identify two 'professional' issues where the lack of a consistent view among clinicians, however trivial or irrelevant they may seem now, caused some confusion for you.

What policies and procedures do you have in your workplace to ensure that these professional issues are not a problem for today's learners? How are the learners made aware of these issues?

If you already have a learner induction programme, check now that these issues are covered. If you do not yet have such a programme, you will have the opportunity to prepare one in Section 11. When you prepare yours, remember to consider if such professional issues are adequately covered.

Summary

In this opening section you have become familiar with the terms that will be used throughout the rest of this pack. You have also considered the position of clinical education within the broader learning process both in general and in light of your own experiences. Subsequent sections will allow you the opportunity to look at each dimension in far greater detail and to consider the development of your own role, where appropriate.

Health and Care Professions Education Forum

The Health Professions Education Forum was established in 1989 as a joint initiative between 10 professions allied to medicine. It is concerned with the 'promotion of effective professional education and training to maintain and develop the highest standards of care for individuals and the community'. Initial membership consisted of: Society of Chiropodists, British Dietetic Association, English National Board for Nursing, Midwifery and Health Visiting, Institute of Medical Laboratory Sciences, College of Occupational Therapists, British Orthoptic Society, Chartered Society of Physiotherapy, British Psychological Society, College of Radiographers, College of Speech and Language Therapists. The Central Council for the Education and Training of Social Workers joined the Forum later, and it has since been known as the Health and Care Professions Education Forum.

Each member organisation maintains a rigorous national overview of its own profession. The Forum broadens this focus to include a perspective of multi-professional healthcare provision in the UK. All members share vital common concerns that standards of care and education should continue to be monitored, maintained and developed. All share an equal appreciation of the need to develop common ground and to explore closer collaboration in education matters in order to meet their own obligations in the light of limitations on resources.

The H&C PEF has an excellent track record in joint working and cooperation between its own members, and also with all parties involved in education and service provision across the UK.

The Forum has held the view that, if the function of education and workforce planning is to be placed at a local level, it will have a detrimental impact on clinical education across the health professions. However, in the absence of any definitive central policy lead, the professions continue to seek to secure their future generations through the development of good-quality clinical education and better-trained, skilled and competent clinical educators.

REFERENCES

Bond C 1990 Personal communication
Brook N 1994 A sharp intake of breath: inspirations in education – some of the issues. Physiotherapy 80(A): 20A–23A
Dawson S 1992 Analysing organisations, 2nd edn. MacMillan Press, London, ch 2, p 32–33
Emery M 1984 Effectiveness of the clinical instructor: students' perspective. Physical Therapy 64(7): 1079–1083
NHS and Community Care Act 1990. HMSO, London
The Chartered Society of Physiotherapy 1991 Curriculum of study. Chartered Society of Physiotherapy, London
Walker A 1991 Clinical education – funding and standards. Physiotherapy 77(11): 742–743

2

The role of the clinical educator

Introduction

The role of the clinical educator is often thought of as having a rather narrow focus and involving merely supervision of the learner. This section sets out to explore and emphasise the diverse nature of what is in fact a multi-faceted role.

Aim

The aim of this section is to encourage you to explore the clinical educator's complex role and to identify aspects of good practice.

Objectives

By the end of this section you should be able to:

1. Identify the role the healthcare professional plays in the workplace as a clinical educator.
2. Analyse the qualities which are needed for the successful fulfilment of this role.

Inherent in the role of all senior healthcare professionals is the responsibility to contribute to the education of the next generation of practitioners. This responsibility can be fulfilled by accepting and assuming the role of the clinical educator and developing the knowledge, attributes, attitudes and skills that are required in this role. These qualities will be considered in greater detail in later sections.

The term 'clinical educator' has already been defined in Section 1 and now needs to be considered in depth.

What aspects do you currently consider this role to include?

Activity 2.1 will help you to consolidate your ideas and to analyse your role as a clinical educator.

ACTIVITY 2.1

This activity should take you no more than 30 minutes.

Conduct a brainstorming session as to the role of the clinical educator. You may work independently, but try to enlist the help of a small group of colleagues (from different disciplines, if possible).

In order to complete this activity successfully you may find it helpful to follow the procedure below:

- ask yourselves the question: 'what is the role of the clinical educator?'
- record the responses on a flipchart or a large sheet of paper
- accept every response at this preliminary stage and do not discuss the various ideas and proposals
- when no more ideas are forthcoming, discuss each response and then organise them into categories.

We undertook this activity ourselves and our results are shown in Figure 2.1.

Now compare the results of your own brainstorming session with ours. You are likely to have additional material to add, as our list is not exhaustive.

Did your list include some of the five main dimensions that we identified as being essential to the clinical educator's role?

Let us now explore these dimensions further.

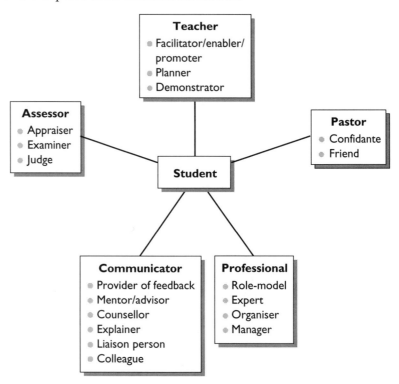

Figure 2.1 The dimensions of the role of the clinical educator

The clinical educator as a teacher/facilitator

This aspect of the role involves the setting of objectives, planning the learning experience and selecting appropriate teaching methods.

The objectives that are set will need to be both realistic and measurable, and there are three types which may be set:

- core placement objectives that relate to the speciality
- local placement objectives that reflect the specific learning opportunities offered by your service
- personal objectives related to the individual's learning needs (these may form the basis of a learning contract, where appropriate; see Section 7).

The core placement objectives are normally set by the learner's host educational institution in close collaboration with representatives from your own clinical speciality. The aim of this is to ensure that both college- and work-based activities are properly integrated and that the requirements of the core curriculum of each of the professional bodies are met. These objectives usually form the basis of the assessment process, which will be considered in detail in Section 8.

In the process of setting objectives, particularly local ones, you will need to take account of what can reasonably be expected of each learner, considering their current stage of academic, personal and professional development.

Box 2.1 gives some examples of core and local objectives for a care of the elderly placement setting.

As a teacher/facilitator, you will also be involved in planning appropriate caseloads for learners and deciding the overall experience they should gain from the placement. To do this you will have to bear in mind each learner's level of entry, i.e. what life experiences they bring to the learning experience, as well as their previous clinical experience.

During the education process you will need to select from a variety of teaching methods – you might tutor learners on a one-to-one basis, for example, or you might teach them in small groups. The method chosen will depend entirely on the learning needs of each individual, on what is required for their professional development and what is appropriate for a particular learning environment.

For further information on teaching and facilitating learning, see Section 7.

Box 2.1 Objectives for a care of the elderly placement

CORE
By the end of the placement the student should be able to:
- demonstrate the ability to select and interpret medical information from notes and X-rays and show how this information is used in assessment
- demonstrate an understanding of the role of the physiotherapist as a member of the multidisciplinary health care team
- communicate effectively and appropriately with (a) patients, their relatives and/or carers; (b) colleagues and other members of the multidisciplinary health care team
- select and demonstrate appropriate examination and assessment procedures
- extract relevant information from patient data and other sources
- identify problems and formulate appropriate objectives of treatment from assessment findings
- apply appropriate treatment techniques efficiently, effectively and safely
- record assessments and treatments given to patients concisely, accurately and neatly as a legal record, using POMR (problem-orientated medical recording)
- demonstrate professionalism in the clinical setting
- demonstrate empathy, understanding and sensitivity in the care and management of the patient
- demonstrate professionalism in the clinical setting
- identify possible areas for personal research

LOCAL
By the end of the placement, the student should be able to:
- discuss the organisation and provision of healthcare for elderly people
- adapt methods of treatment to home environment where necessary
- evaluate and assess treatments given to elderly people
- discuss multiple pathologies and other issues relating to the elderly

---

The clinical educator as a communicator

It is essential for a clinical educator to have excellent communication and associated interpersonal skills. When planning the delivery and evaluation of patient care, you will also be interacting with learners in a constructive and supportive manner. It is important that they should be stimulated and encouraged to contribute at all times in the clinical setting, and that their contribution should be valued.

In addition, you will need to initiate and support a programme of integration and collaboration between the learners and qualified practitioners from your own discipline as well as with other members of the multidisciplinary healthcare team.

You will note that, since communication is considered so vital to the educator's role, reference is made to it throughout later sections.

The clinical educator as an assessor

In your role you will be expected to participate in the assessment of learners by continuously appraising the development of their clinical abilities. This will involve judging each learner's qualities against expected clinical performance and may include a formal assessment of their competence within the clinical setting. The results of any assessments must be communicated both to the learner and to representatives of their host institution.

The issue of assessment is a large and complex topic which will be addressed in detail in Section 8.

The clinical educator as a pastor

For the learner assigned to your area, you may be the only person in the workplace environment to whom they can initially relate. The implication of this is that you may be regarded as a friend, guide or confidante (or all of these) and as such may be required to offer academic and/or personal support to the learner at various times during their placement. On occasions, you may find that there is a conflict between this and other aspects of your role. This is particularly relevant if a learner experiences personal problems whilst on placement with you. In such situations you will need listening and counselling skills. It is always important to acknowledge that counselling is a specialist skill, and for more complex problems it might be necessary for you to seek guidance from the host institution or from a professional counsellor, as appropriate. You may not be able (or willing) to provide the level of support that is required. In such a situation it is worth noting that educational institutions normally provide professional counselling facilities for both full- and part-time learners.

The clinical educator as a professional

As a member of a health profession you are already required to apply professional rules of conduct and standards of good practice to your own working environment. As such, you will be an important role model for the learner. This 'learning by example' is one of the most significant aspects of the transition process from learner to qualified practitioner.

As part of this professional 'socialisation' you will normally help the learner to develop skills for managing their workload.

You will always need to be re-evaluating your own professional practice in order to demonstrate to the learner the value of reflective practice, thus reinforcing your status as a role model.

A major part of your professional role in relation to a learner will be to construct and deliver an appropriate workplace learning programme. This should include the management of all organisational and administrative components of the placement, e.g. timetabling, patient workload etc., and liaison with the learner and other parties. At the same time you will have to be responsive to any changing circumstances in the workplace, such as staff sickness, patient caseloads and other service demands, which may directly or indirectly impact on the learner's placement experience (for further details, see Section 6).

Rewards for the clinical educator

We should not leave our exploration of the educator's role without considering some of the rewards that this role can bring. Gwyer (1993) considered these in a study carried out in the United States. The following tangible rewards were rated as being very important by the respondents in the study.

'To teach learners I must keep my knowledge and skills up to date.'

'Interaction with the learner causes me to constantly analyse the care I'm giving my patients.'

'The learners stimulate me to learn more.'

'I enjoy teaching one-to-one.'

There may also be benefits for the educator's clinical workplace, for example by increased recruitment and heightened national profile as a clinical educational centre. In addition, the professional profiles of the clinical educators themselves may also be enhanced.

As mentioned previously, the role of the clinical educator is multi-faceted and as such requires many different qualities. It is interesting to examine what importance the learner attaches to the elements of the educator's role that we have identified.

ACTIVITY 2.2

This activity is in four parts. Spend no longer than 10 minutes on the first part, 30 minutes on the second part, 15 minutes on the third, 40 minutes on the fourth and 30 minutes on the fifth.

Part 1: Below is a list of 43 characteristics which may be attributed to a clinical educator, based on work by Emery (1984) who identified them and placed them into broad categories. Rank the categories in terms of importance, in your own opinion. For example, if you feel that 'teaching behaviours' is the most important set of characteristics, put number 1 against that. If you feel that 'professional skills behaviours' is the next most important, put number 2 against that, and so on.

CLINICAL INSTRUCTOR BEHAVIOURS

■ **Communication behaviours**
   1. Makes himself/herself understood

2. Provides useful feedback
3. Is an active listener
4. Provides positive feedback on performance
5. Communicates in a non-threatening manner
6. Openly and honestly reveals perceptions held of the learner
7. Provides timely feedback
8. Is open in discussing issues with the learner
9. Teaches in an interactive way; encourages dialogue
10. Provides feedback in private

■ Interpersonal relations behaviours
1. Establishes an environment in which the learner feels comfortable
2. Provides appropriate support for the learner's concerns, frustrations and anxieties
3. Empathises with the learner
4. Demonstrates a genuine concern for patients
5. Introduces the learner to others as a professional
6. Demonstrates a positive regard for the learner as a person

■ Professional skills behaviours
1. Employs physical therapy practice with competence
2. Demonstrates professional behaviour as a member of the healthcare team
3. Demonstrates systematic approach to problem solving
4. Explains physiological basis of physical therapy treatment
5. Explains physiological basis of physical therapy evaluation
6. Demonstrates the appropriate role of physical therapy as part of total healthcare
7. Serves as an appropriate role model
8. Manages own time well
9. Demonstrates leadership among peers

■ Teaching behaviours
1. Allows the learner progressive, appropriate independence
2. Is available to the learner
3. Makes the formal evaluation a constructive process
4. Makes an effective learning experience out of situations as they arise
5. Plans effective learning experiences
6. Provides a variety of patients
7. Questions/coaches in such a way as to help the learner to learn
8. Points out discrepancies in the learner's performance
9. Provides unique learning experiences
10. Demonstrates the relationship between academic knowledge and clinical practice
11. Is accurate in documenting learner evaluation
12. Helps the learner to define specific objectives for the clinical education experience
13. Observes performance in a discreet manner
14. Schedules regular meetings with the learner
15. Plans learning experiences before the learner arrives
16. Manages the learner's time well
17. Is timely in documenting the learner's evaluation
18. Is perceived as a consistent extension of the academic programme

Part 2: Seek the involvement of a colleague or learner and repeat the exercise in Part 1. Their comments will be interesting. Are there any differences in the perspectives of teachers and learners? Emery (1984) found that there were.

Results of this study demonstrated that all behaviours were perceived as

> *somewhat significant and frequent. The learners scored communication as most important followed by interpersonal relations, teaching and professional skills behaviours . . .*
> (Emery 1984)
>
> Bear in mind that a large sample of respondents, such as that used by Emery (1984) who carried out an extensive study in the United States, is required to obtain reliable results.
>
> Part 3: Now consider your own interpretation of the importance of these behaviours in light of your past experience.
>
> Part 4: We recommend that you now read the whole of the Emery (1984) article (see Reader, p.7).
>
> Part 5: A recent study by Cross (1995) compared, in terms of behaviours, the perceptions of the ideal clinical educator held by learners, clinical educators and academic tutors. Interestingly, Cross found that the academic tutors' perceptions were different from those of the learners and the clinical educators. Read the Cross (1995) article (see Reader, p.12) and try to discover why these differences may have occurred.

Let us now consider how you feel the behaviours of the clinical educator can influence learning.

In the next activity we encourage you to refer to your own past experience as a learner.

ACTIVITY 2.3

Spend about 15 minutes on this activity.

Recall three examples of experiences in your own clinical education, at either pre- or post-registration stage, which you feel had a positive effect on any aspect of your learning. Repeat the exercise, but this time consider experiences which you feel had a negative effect on your learning process.

Do you feel that any of these experiences have contributed to the development of your clinical educator's skills, whether highly or poorly developed?

The following direct quotes from learners, which were made after they had been on clinical placements, illustrate how influential the clinical educator's behaviour can be on the learning process.

> *'When discussing patient management, I was praised and encouraged if my understanding was good. If it wasn't good, I was encouraged to read books, notes, ask questions, etc. I was never harshly criticised but guided and corrected.'*

> *'It was made perfectly clear that they were surprised by my lack of knowledge. I was constantly compared with learners who had previously been there on placement. I was told that my attitude was 'student-like' and unprofessional. This made me nervous, as I was unsure what I was doing wrong and unable to discuss it as I was too upset. It also made me paranoid as I didn't know who had said this about me and what I had done to deserve it.'*

You may have encountered an educator whose approach you did not benefit from.

Davis & McKain (1975) emphasise how important it is for educators to be self-aware and to recognise their own 'faults', which they call 'not OK' behaviours. They see this self-awareness as being critical to the clinical educator's role as a teacher and 'developer of behaviour'.

The next activity helps you to explore 'not OK' behaviours in more detail and will also help you to develop your own self-awareness.

ACTIVITY 2.4

Read the article by Davis & McKain (1975) (see Reader, p. 20) now and list any 'OK' and 'not OK' behaviours you feel might feature in your role as a clinical educator.

Summary

In this section we have considered the complex multi-faceted role of the clinical educator and explored the major dimensions of this role as a:

- teacher
- communicator
- assessor
- pastor
- professional.

Now complete the following reflective exercise to assess what you have learned having worked through this section.

SUMMARY ACTIVITY

Imagine you are preparing for your first experience as a clinical educator. Evaluate the personal qualities that you will bring to this new situation and identify behaviours that you would wish to enhance.

We hope that by continuing to work through this package, it will enable you to recognise your strengths as a clinical educator and will assist you to enhance the behaviours you have addressed in the previous reflective exercise.

REFERENCES

Cross V 1995 Perceptions of the ideal clinical educator in physiotherapy education. Physiotherapy 81(9): 506–513

Davis C M, McKain A E 1975 Clinical education: awareness of our 'not-OK' behaviour. Physical Therapy 55(5): 505–506

Emery M J 1984 Effectiveness of the clinical instructor: students' perspective. Physical Therapy 64(7): 1079–1083

Gwyer J 1993 Rewards of teaching physical therapy students: clinical instructor's perspective. Journal of Physical Therapy Education 7(2): 63–66

3

Identifying the learner and educator and their interactions

Introduction

Having investigated the multi-faceted role of the clinical educator in the last section, we are now going to look at the players in the educational setting in more detail. We will also consider the ways in which these players interact.

Aim

The aim of this section is to enable you to identify who the learners are in the clinical education setting, and to explore some of the characteristics of educators and learners, and the relationships they have with each other.

Objectives

By the end of this section you should be able to:

1. Identify groups of learners with whom you may work in the clinical setting.
2. Discuss the characteristics of learners and teachers/educators.
3. Appreciate the different ways in which learners and educators interact.
4. Demonstrate an awareness of the differences in the ways that learners and educators store and utilise information.

Identifying the learner

A learner can be defined as 'a person who is gaining knowledge, skills or attitudes by study or experience or by being taught'.

In many ways this definition is acceptable but it has its limitations. The term 'taught' is probably misleading as it implies that the learner has a very passive role. It gives the impression that knowledge is imparted to the passive recipient by a teacher who expects, and is expected, to be the sole source of that knowledge. This overly instructive or didactic approach may be familiar to you from learning experiences in your past, in which case you can probably pinpoint aspects of this approach that you found unsatisfactory and others that were satisfactory.

ACTIVITY 3.1

This activity should take no longer than 20 minutes.

Discuss your experiences of didactic teaching with some of your colleagues. Note down positive and negative statements that are made. Keep this list, as it will be useful to reflect on it again in Section 11.

Many of us identify the typical teacher/learner situation as that which occurs between a learner health professional and a qualified health professional (the clinical educator). It is, however, highly likely that the clinical educator will be involved in a much broader spectrum of teacher/learner situations during the course of their professional life.

ACTIVITY 3.2

Spend no longer than 10 minutes on this activity.

Think carefully about the educator/learner interactions that you and/or your colleagues are regularly involved in. Identify who the learners are, and in each case state the purpose of the learning activity.

Your list of learners may include doctors, nurses, occupational therapists, podiatrists, radiographers, speech and language therapists, ancillary workers, carers, general public, patients, workers in industry and members of your own professional group. When identifying the purposes of the learning activities, you may have included, for example, health education, patient education, education of other healthcare professionals and back care for industrial workers.

It is useful to think of the clinical setting, where a learner is gaining clinical experience alongside an experienced therapist (the educator), as one which involves a triangular relationship between the educator, the learner and the patient undergoing treatment. All three parties will learn from each other, and at the same time contribute to each other's learning process, during different stages of the clinical interaction. This makes the clinical setting a very dynamic educational environment.

It is difficult to imagine a clinical interaction in which the clinician does not ultimately take on a teaching role and the patient take on the role of a learner. It may be that you take your role in relation to this group of learners for granted. You may in fact find that many of the skills you have developed in this type of interaction can be transferred to contacts with other learners. Equally, it is likely that new skills you develop in relation to learners can be incorporated into the teaching role you adopt with patients or other groups previously identified.

Having identified learners with whom you work in the clinical setting, let us now consider the differences that might exist among them. There may be differences between learners within the same group, as well as between learners belonging to different groups.

Differences among learners

Let us look at the learner more closely. According to Whitcomb (1992) learners vary in many ways, for example in their interests, needs and capacities. There are also differences in their abilities to learn and the rates at which they learn. It is important that, as a clinical educator, you are able to acknowledge and respond to these differences. The learner must be considered not just as a thinking person, but also as a feeling individual who is able to carry out physical tasks – as Whitcomb says, 'a feeling and doing as well as a thinking person'. There are other ways in which learners vary and which may have a direct influence on their learning, for example personality factors, age, gender, cultural background and prior learning achievements (Stenglehoffen 1993). Again, it is important that the educator is able to recognise these variables and their possible implications. Some of these factors will be given greater consideration in Section 5.

The educator identified

Many people perform educational roles in both formal and informal contexts (Knowles 1980). Yet not all educators undergo a formal training. It could be said that anyone who helps another person to learn is an educator.

ACTIVITY 3.3

Earlier in this section you identified learner/educator interactions that you and/or your colleagues are involved in. Review this list, highlighting the various ways in which you as a health professional help other people to learn, i.e. the many contexts in which you should be regarded as an educator.

We have already discussed the role of the clinical educator in Section 2. Knowles (1980) has highlighted two key dimensions of this role which have implications for the individuals involved:

1. it is principally the role of an educator of adults
2. it is performed in an interpersonal setting which is multidimensional.

The implications of these dimensions for the individual will be discussed in Sections 4 and 6.

Best (1988) believes that health professionals have varying perceptions of the task of clinical education. These perceptions are influenced by their own learner experiences of clinical education, their work situations, their more recent experiences of learner contact, their stage of professional development and their own intrinsic personal needs. In turn these perceptions will colour the educator's attitude towards learners.

Teaching and learning

As has been seen, there is considerable diversity both within a single group of learners and among different groups of learners. In addition to this, the perceptions of the role of the educator, as held by the educators themselves, vary widely. This is true even for individual educators, whose perceptions of the role change at different stages in their careers. All of these variations in individuals come together in the clinical setting and this cocktail of assorted variables within a clinical education setting is highly potent, creating at times a very fruitful and stimulating interaction between learner and educator. Sadly, however, there are also times when it can be highly explosive and destructive.

Now that the key players in clinical education have been introduced, let us explore the concept of learning and how it influences educator/learner interaction.

Watts (1990) defines learning in two ways:

1. Learning is the acquisition of knowledge through instruction.
2. Learning is a change in behaviour that results from experience.

These two definitions indicate two very different approaches to education. The first implies a content-centred, educator-initiated approach. In other words, the educator chooses the information to be covered and decides how to present it so that it is easily absorbed by the learner. In this case, the learner acts as a passive receptacle for knowledge, which is heavily prescribed by the educator.

The second definition concentrates attention on the learner and how their memory, judgments, beliefs and actions are shaped by events in which they take an active part. In this context, learners are given an opportunity actually to try out the behaviours they seek to learn. They are then guided through the experience in such a way that desirable changes in their performance are achieved (Watts 1990). Watts felt that these two approaches to education often occur in tandem. She considered that the purpose of education is to help learners to change, but recognised that providing information is one of the things that educators must do in order to make changes in behaviour possible.

ACTIVITY 3.4

Spend no longer than 1 hour on this activity.

Read the extract 'The events of learning and functions of teaching' taken from Watts (1990) (see Reader, p. 22).

Think about how the information given in this extract might affect the way you structure a learner's period of clinical education experience.

It appears that we learn best when things have meaning, and that the learning process is stimulated when the how and why are known. For example, when junior staff members attempt to understand the concept of a clinical audit, the process of understanding is made much easier if an insight has already been gained into what quality is, how it can be measured, and to whom quality of care is important. Likewise, when a learner is introduced to the topic of infection control, it is difficult to comprehend the rationale behind it without an understanding of how infection is produced, how it spreads and why certain individuals are more susceptible to infection than others.

Interest is also an important factor in learning. New interests usually grow out of old interests. Learning occurs largely in terms of past experience and through association – hence the value of helping the learner to create a rich background of experience.

Satisfaction is another factor to consider. We learn more rapidly when it gives us satisfaction. It is therefore important that tasks are kept within the learner's educational experience and maturity, i.e. at the right level. Learners need guidance from educators in maintaining aspirations that are consistent with what they can achieve (Whitcomb 1992). The learning process is always enhanced if it is made as pleasant and as enjoyable as possible, but obviously this must occur without compromising standards of patient care.

Learning, then, is a process of experiencing, reacting and doing. We learn by listening, visualising, recalling, memorising, reasoning, judging and thinking, and generally speaking, the more active the learner is in the process, the more effective their learning will be. Encouragement to participate is therefore vital. In terms of clinical education, Skully & Shepherd (1983) defined the process as a dynamic enabling process, in which the learner is helped by a clinical educator to make the best use of their knowledge and skills in the effort to improve their abilities. In this way the job is completed more effectively and with increasing satisfaction for the learners, their clinical educator, their profession and their host-educational institution. Yonke (1979) described clinical education as an interactive process where there is difficulty in separating teaching from learning and in which the learner/educator relationship dramatically affects the learner's learning and subsequent performance.

Wong & Wong (1980) considered that this relationship is always significant and that learners and educators continually interact together, with both positive and negative outcomes. The individual personalities, perceptions and needs of the educator and learner can often vary enormously. As a result, they can both sometimes find the interaction process difficult, especially if a 'personality clash' arises. Although this might happen with a particular educator and learner, it is the case that, given the same set of circumstances and setting, but with a different learner or educator, the resulting experience could be both stimulating and rewarding for all participants.

Other differences arise between the educator (expert) and the learner (novice), for example in the ways they store and use information. Learners see items in isolation and can only cope with small pieces of information. Experts appear to organise the small pieces of information into chunks which are then stored in their long-term memory. Often educators expect learners to arrive at the same conclusions as they do without taking into account these differences in processing (Edding 1987).

Here is a typical example of how educators and learners store and use information in different ways. It occurs frequently in the clinical examination setting. Consider an examination of a patient suffering from lumbar spine dysfunction. The clinician who is performing the examination will previously have stored information about the anatomy of the spine, the physiological function of the spinal joints and the relevant examination procedures, and will also have learned about various pathologies which might affect the spine. These chunks of information will have been organised into a cohesive whole. This clinician is now able to relate subjective data gained during the examination of the patient to their physical findings and thus arrive at a relevant and accurate clinical orthopaedic diagnosis. For the learner, however, this is a much more difficult process. They may know the anatomy of the spine and the physiology of spinal joint function and they may have knowledge of the relevant examination procedures, but they will probably lack the ability early in their careers to link their examination findings to the anatomy, physiology and pathology of the patient. It is therefore much more difficult for the learner to make an accurate and clear-cut diagnosis in this situation than it is for the experienced clinician. This aquisition of knowledge and its application is considered in Section 8 in relation to Bloom's (1956) Taxonomy of Learning.

The clinical education setting is a most complex laboratory for the learner. In this laboratory, they must learn to integrate prior theoretical knowledge and practical skills, while taking on board new knowledge, modifying existing practical skills and acquiring new skills. At the same time, they must attempt to relate on a personal level to patients from varied social backgrounds with multiple physical and possibly psycho-social problems; to their clinical educator; and on occasions to visiting members of academic staff from host educational institutions. This exercise is no mean feat, even for the expert, and thus for the learner it is a potentially highly stressful situation which can have a detrimental effect on the total learning experience.

Within the educator/learner relationship, consensus must be reached that the patient has to come first and that all learner-related activities must occur within this context. There is therefore a potential conflict between the educator's responsibility for the learner and their learning and the ethical responsibility for patient care.

Best's (1988) adaption of a management grid demonstrates the possible interactions between the educator and the learner. It is designed to show the balance between the educator's concern for the learner and concern for learner productivity, i.e. the numbers of patients treated.

ACTIVITY 3.5

Spend about 1 hour on this activity.

Read the section on the 'Adaption of a managerial grid for clinical supervision' from Best's (1988) article (see Reader, p. 30).

Use the grid to identify and demonstrate the balance that you maintain in the relationship between your concern for the learner and your concern for physiotherapy tasks.

Also when reading the extract, explore the idea of maternalistic/paternalistic supervisory input. This is where the clinical educator takes complete responsibility for an individual's learning and experiences, allowing the learner to become dependent on them and hindering creativity and independence.

Summary

In this section, we have investigated the breadth of teacher/learner situations in which the clinical educator may participate during their professional life. We have explored the variations which can exist among learners. We have identified the educator and highlighted how perceptions of the task of clinical education can vary among educators themselves. We have explored the concept of learning and how it influences educator/learner interactions, and we have examined some of the differences between learners and educators, and how these differences can influence the learner/educator relationship.

Finally, we have introduced the idea of maternalistic/paternalistic supervisory input and discussed how the balance that you maintain in the relationship between your concern for the learner and your concern for physiotherapy tasks determines the quality of learning that will be experienced by the learners for whom you have responsibility.

SUMMARY ACTIVITY

Consider carefully your perception of the role of the clinical educator and the educator/learner relationship. Having identified in activity 3.5 the balance that you maintain in the relationship between your concern for the learner and your concern for physiotherapy tasks, consider now whether you may need to modify your approach to the task of clinical education in the future in order to ensure that learners will obtain maximum benefit from your input as an educator.

Now that you have considered the learner and the educator in more depth, let us consider the educational theories which relate to the concept of learning.

REFERENCES

Best D 1988 Physiotherapy clinical supervision effectiveness and use of models. Australian Journal of Physiotherapy 34(4): 209–214

Bloom B 1956 Taxonomy of educational objectives: the classification of educational goals. Handbook 1 – Cognitive domain. McKay, New York

Edding T 1987 Clinical problem solving in physical therapy and its implications for curriculum development. Proceedings of the 10th International Congress of the World Confederation for Physical Therapy, Book 1. World Confederation of Physical Therapists, Sidney, p 100–104

Knowles M S 1980 The modern process of adult education, 2nd edn. Association Press, Chicago

Skully R, Shepherd K 1983 Clinical teaching in physical therapy education. Physical Therapy 63(3): 349–358

Stenglehoffen J 1993 Teaching students in clinical settings. Chapman and Hall, London, p 55–57

Watts N 1990 Handbook of clinical teaching. Churchill Livingstone, Edinburgh, p 5–12

Whitcombe B 1992 Methods of clinical instruction in physical therapy. Physical Therapy Review 31(4): 129–134

Wong S, Wong J 1980 The effectiveness of clinical teaching: a model for self evaluation. Journal of Advanced Nursing 5: 531–537

Yonke A 1979 The art and science of clinical teaching. Medical Education 13: 86–90

4

Learning theories

Introduction

Both educators and learners should understand the processes and characteristics that are associated with successful learning. As partners and participants in the learning process, they will then be equipped to fulfil their respective roles. When educators appreciate that people have different learning styles and strategies, and that motivation to learn can vary greatly between individuals, then teaching is more effective and learning is enhanced. When educators reflect on their own learning experiences and integrate the principles of adult learning theory into their thinking, they should find themselves better able to relate to the needs of students and junior colleagues.

With these ideas in mind, questions as to how and why adults learn are explored in this section.

Aim

The aim of this section is to introduce some key concepts of contemporary adult learning theory and to encourage you to explore their relevance to the process of clinical education and learning.

Objectives

By the end of this section you should be able to:

1. Describe and discuss the characteristics that are associated with adult learners.
2. Appreciate some of the individual differences in adult learning styles and strategies.
3. Appreciate the importance of motivation to learn and consider how motivation can be maximised.
4. Discuss the relevance of adult learning theories to teaching and learning in the clinical setting.

ACTIVITY 4.1

This activity should take at least 30 minutes. It should provide a useful framework within which to explore your own style and approach to learning. Record your responses so that you will be able to refer to them easily as you work through this section.

Think of a continuing professional education course the content of which is directly applicable to your personal and professional development in your current clinical role. This is likely to be a course that you hope to follow in the future. Now do the following:

- Name this course so that this activity has direct relevance to you and the planning of your continuing education programme.
- State explicitly:
  - why you are applying to do this course
  - what you feel you will bring to the course
  - what you hope to gain from the course.
- Describe how you will prepare yourself prior to the start of the course.
- Describe how you will approach in-course activities and assignments.
- State which activities you are especially looking forward to.

Keep your responses close to hand as you work through this section.

Adults as learners

Individuals embarking on higher and professional education are all adult learners. Although many will have come to college or university straight from school with less 'life experience' than so-called 'mature' learners, all of them will bring a wealth of past experience in relation to teaching and learning. This experience will have influenced and shaped their attitudes and approaches to learning. Knowles (1983) suggests that there is a subtle difference between the ways in which children and adults regard their experiences.

To a child, an experience is something that happens to him; it is an external event that affects him, not an integral part of him. If you ask a child who he is, he is likely to answer in terms of who his parents are, who his older brothers and sisters are, what street he lives on and what school he attends. His self-identity is largely derived from external sources.

But to an adult his experience is him. He defines who he is, establishes his self-identity, in terms of his accumulation of a unique set of experiences. So if you ask an adult who he is, he is likely to identify himself in terms of what his occupation is, where he has worked, where he has travelled, what his training and experience have equipped him to do, and what his achievements have been. An adult is what he has done. (Knowles 1983, p.61)

Knowles believes that relating new learning to existing experience is a key feature of the adult learning process.

Background to Knowles' theory of adult learning

Knowles's theory is based on four primary assumptions about adults as learners:

1. they see themselves as self-directing and responsible
2. they possess an accumulation of experience which is a resource for their own learning and that of others
3. they are motivated to learn when they perceive the activity as being directly related to their own 'life tasks'
4. their interests tend to focus on problem-solving rather than on abstract content or theory.

ACTIVITY 4.2

Do you agree with the characteristics of adult learners that Knowles has identified? Return to the notes you made during Activity 4.1. Are any of the characteristics he identifies evident in your account of how you intend to approach the continuing education programme?

Conditions for 'superior' teaching and learning

The learning environment must have the following characteristics. It should be physically comfortable, there should be mutual trust and respect, mutual helpfulness, freedom of expression and an acceptance of differences. So important is it to have a favourable learning environment, that a whole section of this package has been dedicated to a discussion of how this might be achieved. In a favourable learning environment, the educator will appreciate that adult learners may face specific challenges associated with taking responsibility for their own learning and becoming self-directing. The following discussion identifies just some of these challenges.

● *Adults may experience shock when first required to participate actively in a learning session and to share responsibility with the teacher for initiating discussions that enhance the acquisition of knowledge and formation of concepts.*

This is especially true if they have come from a 'traditional' educational background, i.e. one in which the teacher always organises and directs the learning experience. In successful clinical education, it is imperative that the learner and the educator approach the challenge of problem-solving together. The clinical educator will act as guide and helper but the learner must be both willing and able to engage in what might be described as 'mutual enquiry'. This is a process in which both learner and educator discuss clinical findings, explore underlying pathology, and propose, test and rationalise appropriate therapeutic intervention.

Learners will often be anxious about expressing their ideas and offering their interpretation of clinical findings when the problems relate to the needs of 'real' patients and clients, and when their colleagues are senior and experienced clinicians. An important role for the college-based educator is to offer learning opportunities that simulate clinical problem-solving in the 'security' of the classroom, away from the responsibilities that come from direct patient contact and clinical work. In this way, when the time comes for this direct contact, learners will be better prepared to participate in problem-solving and treatment planning. These activities require the clinician to integrate examination and assessment processes, subsequent findings and patient evaluation, and as such demand high levels of intellect and sophisticated approaches to learning.

● *Learners must be prepared to accept the learning experience as belonging to them; its goals must be relevant to their particular learning needs.*

Clearly, the ability to identify personal objectives is important. At the beginning of the placement, in an induction interview, the clinical educator and the learner should work together to tailor the learning experience to the learner's specific needs and begin work on developing a learning contract. This important preliminary stage of the placement will be discussed fully in Chapter 10, which addresses the setting of objectives.

● *Learners must accept a share of the responsibility for planning and managing a learning experience and should participate actively in all stages of the process.*

The educator constantly supports this activity by making use of the learner's experience and nurturing a sense of progress towards the identified goals.

ACTIVITY 4.3

Refer again to the plans you made during Activity 4.1 concerning the continuing education course. Is there any evidence from your notes that you face challenges that have been presented as specific to adult learners?

Are you likely to draw upon Knowles' theories when you are working with learners in the future and helping them to plan their clinical learning experiences?

More about adult learning theory and its relationship with other schools of thought

Knowles' concept of adult learning spans several broad categories (or 'schools') of learning theory, according to Mast & Van Atta (1986, p. 3).

It acknowledges the values of **reinforcement** *and* **social learning** *as did the behaviourists (e.g. Skinner (1953) and Bandura (1963)); it stresses* **individual differences** *within general stages or* **levels of learning** *as did Piaget (1958) or Gagne (1975), and others of the so-called* **cognitive** *school; and it emphasises* **self-determination, self-assessment and the involvement of the whole person** *in the learning process as did* **humanists** *such as Maslow (1943) and Rogers (1983).* (Mast & Van Atta 1986, p. 3)

ACTIVITY 4.4

Below are two articles which apply some of the learning theories mentioned above. They are included in your Reader (pp 36 & 42).

1. Coulter M A 1990 A review of two theories of learning and their application in the practice of nurse education. Nurse Education Today 10: 333-338
2. Hulse S F 1992 Learning theories: something for everyone. Radiologic Technology 63(3): 198-202

Select one of these which stimulates your interest and read it carefully.

How relevant would the concepts outlined in the article be if you were embarking on your chosen continuing education course?

In your opinion, how relevant to the process of clinical education are these concepts?

You may also wish to follow up on one of the 'schools' of learning theory. These will be discussed in both psychology and educational theory texts.

Individuality and learning styles

It is very important for educators to acknowledge that learners are individuals who have preferred styles for both teaching and learning. Jobling (1987) discussed some of the reasons for these differences between learners and their implications for educating and learning.

ACTIVITY 4.5

Please read Jobling (1987) now (see Reader, p. 47).

Do you tend to select teaching methods consistent with your own preferred learning styles?

Can you remember ever having difficulty responding to a particular teaching style?

What was the outcome of that experience for you as a learner?

Taking responsibility for learning – are self-directed or self-initiated learning strategies the answer?

Knowles (1983) suggested that self-directed learning involves learners identifying their own learning needs, establishing goals, deciding on what learning activities will take place, and assessing and evaluating success for themselves.

The teacher's or educator's role is one of enabling this learning to take place. This means, in essence, a relationship where the learner 'decides' and the teacher 'responds'. This relationship, in its purest state, might be suitable in less formal and discovery-orientated approaches, but where the learning outcome is dictated by statute and where professional core curricula are concerned, there must be some measure of control. One also has to consider time implications, particularly in the clinical environment, as well as keeping both ethical issues and the importance of the patient's needs to the fore. However, the use of adult learning principles (andragogic) should predominate over the use of 'pedagogic' techniques, which have been developed as a result of experience and research related to the teaching of children.

One way of reconciling issues of learner and educator control is to introduce learning 'themes', e.g. 'goal setting', 'prioritisation of needs' and 'utilisation of examination and assessment findings'. These can be approached by assisting the learner to draw up learning contracts relating to these essential components of the clinical learning experience. Thus there is direction given to both the learning process and outcome, but the needs, wishes and individuality of the learner are integrated and respected (for further detail on learning contracts see Section 7).

A partnership model of self-directed learning has been recommended by Slevin & Lavery (1991). In Table 4.1 they illustrate how control might be shared by the learner and the teacher.

These authors highlight the need for supervisory sessions to be learning-orientated. In other words, the learner should have the opportunity to present ongoing work and explain any difficulties. The educator should provide guidance and direction as appropriate and give the learner feedback on progress. It is important to give positive reinforcement as often as possible. It is also desirable to avoid didactic (over-instructive) approaches. In this way, independent learning behaviours are nurtured in a supportive climate.

In this context, it is also important to acknowledge that, at the pre-registration level, healthcare professional courses cannot furnish learners with everything they are going to need for a lifetime's career. This statement may seem obvious. However, all too frequently professional educators, both college- and clinically based, overload learners with information in an attempt to bring them up to their own level of competence and skill. Senior professionals with a wealth of clinical experience sometimes find it difficult to remember what it was like to function

Table 4.1 Control in the partnership of self-directed study

Stage	Control of learning	
	Student	Teacher
Identification of learning needs	Higher • individual needs outlined	Lower • needs related to programme requirements
Statement of objectives/specification of learning outcomes	Lower • viewed in context of previous learning and felt need	Higher • learning outcomes as specified in statutory instruments must be met
Programme planning	Equal • negotiated learning contract	Equal • negotiated learning contract
Learning activities	Higher • commitment to agreed programme and contracted to achieve learning outcomes	Lower • commitment to facilitating, advising, guiding, resourcing and monitoring progress
Evaluation	Equal • self-assessment	Equal • teacher assessment

professionally without their current level of expertise. As a result, they find it hard to relate to the needs of a learner. Their expectations of learners may therefore be inappropriate or unrealistic. They may attempt to 'compensate' for the learner's 'lack of knowledge' by attempting constantly to 'top up' their knowledge base. However, most of the time they will simply impart information, with the learner in the role of passive recipient. This type of approach can actually compromise the learner's personal and professional development. Unless learners are actively involved in seeking knowledge, and understanding and processing information, then there are no guarantees that because the teacher has taught, the learner has learned! This is one of the most powerful arguments for encouraging self-directed learning behaviours. The foundations must be laid for a career of continuing professional development, and college- and clinically based educators share the responsibility for doing this.

However, in 1987, Titchen alerted physiotherapy educators to the fact that practising therapists were not very proficient at undertaking self-initiated learning. Present-day educators may well argue that the advent of undergraduate courses has addressed many of the issues raised by Titchen (1987).

ACTIVITY 4.6

Please read Titchen's (1987) article now (see Reader, p. 51).

How far do you consider that the issues raised by Titchen have been addressed in contemporary clinical educational practice?

Courses that promote self-directed and self-responsible learning behaviours

Healthcare professional education programmes must be validated by both the educational institution and the appropriate professional bodies. Course teams engage in detailed educational planning and are required to submit full documentation of their course plans in order to fulfil the requirements of the validation process. Course programmes that actively encourage the development of self-directed learning will declare an allegiance to such principles in their philosophical statements, course aims and objectives. In selecting and organising the content of the course programme, the way in which healthcare professional knowledge changes over time will be taken into account. Many authors have argued that the knowledge gained by healthcare professional learners at university could well be obsolete within as little as 5 years. Hence, there is a commitment to developing:

- self-responsible learning strategies
- flexibility and adaptability of both mind and attitude
- commitment to life-long learning
- research awareness and skill.

These are preferred to the mere transmission and assimilation of information. Neame & Powis (1981) discussed this issue in relation to medical education and link self-directed learning behaviours and accountability to the needs of the healthcare consumer:

> *. . . the practitioner must be able to review and update his practices regularly if his livelihood and the health of his patients are not to be affected adversely.*
> (Neame & Powis 1981, p. 886)

In courses that promote self-directed and self-responsible learning behaviours, the range of teaching and learning methods utilised should reflect strategies which help the learner to take responsibility for their own learning, e.g. assisted independent study, self-instructional materials, guided study and the negotiation of learning contracts. College-based educators and their clinical colleagues will discuss how such approaches may be extended to the clinical setting so as best to integrate theoretical knowledge and practice. The completed course document will describe a curriculum which moves progressively towards learner-centred learning, i.e. the emphasis is ultimately on what the learner learns and not on what the teacher teaches. Naturally, the earlier in the course the activity occurs, the more it will tend to be under the teacher's control. However, from a very early stage, active learning activities running in parallel to the more formal or didactic approaches will encourage the learners to become more self-directed. This approach will be used in both teaching and assessment.

ACTIVITY 4.7

Obtain a copy of the full course document for one course programme followed by learners on placement at your clinical area.

What evidence can you find of the promotion of self-directed learning behaviours? Does the wording of the course objectives suggest that this aim is promoted?

How far is this approach encouraged and facilitated in the clinical education programme? Is the approach explicit in the handbooks circulated to clinical educators?

The philosophy of learners taking responsibility for their own learning has been strongly supported here. However, individuals will approach this challenge in many different ways. The rest of this section will explore learning styles and strategies and their relevance to clinical education.

Analysing learning

We all have learning styles which suit us as individuals. They relate to the way in which we approach study as well as to the way we think. Learning styles are related to personality and have nothing to do with intelligence. In the clinical setting where teaching often takes place on an individual basis or in a small group, the teacher and the learner interact very closely. If the educator's teaching style and the learner's learning style are incompatible, there will be a potential source of tension.

Research has shown that there are four main learning styles. Various characteristics are associated with each of these styles. Honey & Mumford (1986) group these characteristics under the headings:

● activist
● reflector
● theorist
● pragmatist.

The characteristics of each type are summarised in Box 4.1 by Stengelhofen (1993).

Box 4.1 Description of learning styles (adapted from Honey & Mumford 1986)

Activists
– involve themselves fully, without bias, in new experiences
– enjoy the here and now, happy to be dominated by immediate experiences
– open-minded, not sceptical
– enthusiastic about anything new
– dash in where angels fear to tread
– like brainstorming problems
– bored with implementation and longer-term consolidation
– gregarious, involve themselves with others
– seek to centre all the activities around them.

Reflectors
– like to stand back to ponder experiences, thoughtful
– observe from many different perspectives
– collect data, chew over before coming to conclusions
– tend to postpone reaching conclusions
– cautious, leave no stone unturned
– prefer to take back seat in meetings and discussions
– enjoy observing people in action
– listen to others
– adopt a low profile
– have a slightly distant, tolerant, unruffled air.

Theorists
– integrate observations into complex, logical theories
– think problems through step-by-step
– assimilate disparate facts into cohesive whole
– tend to be perfectionists
– like to analyse
– tend to feel uncomfortable with subjective judgments
– tend to be detached, analytical and rational.

Pragmatists
– keen on trying out ideas, theories and techniques
– positively search out new ideas
– like to experiment
– like to get on with things and act quickly
– tend to be impatient with lengthy open-ended discussion
– essentially practical, like making practical decisions
– respond to problems and opportunities as a challenge.

ACTIVITY 4.8

Read the description of Honey & Mumford's learning styles (Box 4.1) and decide which category you would place yourself in. If you have a learner on placement with you or if you are responsible for a junior member of staff, ask them to do likewise.

It is also important for educators to reflect on their predominant teaching characteristics. Stengelhofen (1993) provides a useful summary of the work of Brasseur & Anderson (1983), which describes direct and indirect teaching styles. They propose that these styles lead to different behaviours in the learner.

ACTIVITY 4.9

Use the summary chart in Box 4.2 to help you identify your predominant teaching styles. How do these relate to the learning styles of your junior colleagues?

Box 4.2 Direct and indirect learning styles (adapted from Brasseur & Anderson 1983)

Direct	Indirect
• Dominated by the supervisor	• More student-centred
	• Supervisor talks less, listens more
• High proportion of supervisor talking, i.e. giving information, giving opinions, giving suggestions, giving criticisms	• Supportive relationship
	• Asks questions
	• Accepts and uses ideas
	• Reflects
	• Summarizes student's ideas and feelings

These styles lead to different behaviours in the learner

Direct style leads to:	*Indirect style leads to:*
• Supervisor control	• Collaborative problem-solving
• Evaluation, supervisor as expert	
Student dependence	**Student independence**

The learner's approach to clinical education and its link with quality of learning outcome

Marton & Saljo (1976) were critical of attempts to describe the outcome of learning in quantitative terms, i.e. to try to calculate how much the learner knows at the end of the placement and how many facts have been assimilated. They described 'levels of processing' information which cover a broad spectrum, from superficial to deep, and involve very different styles and approaches. They highlighted the importance of understanding the different ways in which a learner might approach the subject matter. They argued that there is a direct relationship between the level of processing and the quality of the learning outcome. 'Deep' levels of processing are said to lead to the attainment of 'concepts'. Concepts enable us to make sense of a complex array of material and information. The formation and utilisation of concepts are important features of healthcare professional practice.

One of the authors of this package conducted a small study which duplicated one of Marton & Saljo's experiments. This study reviewed the strategic approaches and consequent learning outcomes of a group of first year physiotherapy students who undertook a reading assignment early on in their course programme. The students were studying the physiology of muscle contraction. After completing their reading assignment, they were asked to write a brief summary of the text and to describe their approach to the reading assignment. The following statements were made by members of the group and demonstrate both 'deep' and 'superficial' approaches.

- *'Deep' approaches*
'I tried to picture the processes as I went along - to see it all working. I spent time relating the text to my diagrams.'

'I was intent on understanding the method of muscle contraction and tried to relate the structure of actin and myosin to concepts of muscle as a contractile tissue.'

'At the end of each section, I ensured that new material was put into perspective and that my new found knowledge "fitted in" . . . finally, structure and function had become very much as one in the overall picture of the text.'

'I managed to pick out the main points and generally understand the mechanisms . . .'

'My mind automatically concentrated on mechanisms – tending to neglect detail of terminology.'

'I tend to grapple with understanding, and leave minute detail to the last minute before exams!'

'I just try to understand, but not to memorise exact details.'

- *'Superficial' approaches*
'I read the book and took notes – there seemed a lot to read and remember.'

'I read through the chapter – bits I had done at A-level. I skipped through very quickly – it was hard to remember without writing simple notes.'

This small study supported Marton & Saljo's conclusions that higher levels of learning outcome were associated with 'deeper' levels of approach to the assignment.

You will have observed that there are a greater number of comments which demonstrate a 'deep' level of processing. This was representative of the group approach and was a very pleasing finding. You would perhaps expect learners who have gained places to study on a healthcare professional course to be capable of such sophisticated approaches to their learning assignments. However, it is worth noting that such findings also indicate that the approach to teaching actually encouraged learners to use their natural abilities and skills.

Sophisticated approaches to learning and the importance of motivation

In the same study, it was interesting, but perhaps not surprising, to find that some students had actually changed their learning strategy since arriving at college. Where such a change had occurred, students indicated that it was due to increased commitment to their learning and the associated increase in motivation. The necessity of a sound knowledge base for effective practice was recognised and acted upon.

'I have much greater interest in physiotherapy . . . I want to learn about it . . . I spend more time . . . I want to understand. I used to skip through reading for A-level.'

'I'm trying to learn for my own benefit – as opposed to my teacher's.'

'I'm taking more notice, showing more interest.'

'I take longer . . . I follow up references . . . I look at lecture notes and other books. I try to learn - not just read 'cos I've been told to.'

'On this course, my approach is different because this is the real thing as far as careers are concerned. Mistakes made now may affect my results in June and therefore my career. Basically, my approach is far more serious, and perhaps, hopefully more mature.'

Summary

These final student's comments indicate that there are strong links between the different ideas associated with contemporary adult learning theories that have been introduced in this chapter, i.e.

- adult learning principles
- learning styles and strategies
- self-directed learning
- 'deep' approaches to the processing of information and their link with the quality of the learning outcome
- the importance of motivation to learn.

We propose that the challenges of clinical education offer opportunities for educators, together with their learners, to explore and utilise adult learning principles. It could be argued that the required outcome of clinical education, i.e. a competent, independent practitioner, actually demands such an approach.

 SUMMARY ACTIVITY

Return to your strategic plans for your continuing education course (Activity 4.1). Make a judgement about the likely quality of your learning outcome based on the evidence of learning styles, approaches and strategies that appear in your notes.

Make a similar judgement about a learner's clinical placement in which you have been involved. Most importantly, think how that learner's efforts and endeavours could have been supported.

REFERENCES

Bandura A, Walters R H 1963 Social learning and personality development. Rinehart and Winston, New York

Brasseur J A , Anderson J L 1983 Observed differences between direct, indirect and direct/indirect video-taped supervisory conferences. Journal of Speech and Hearing Research 26: 344–355

Coulter M A 1990 A review of two theories of learning and their application in the practice of nurse education. Nurse Education Today 10: 333–338

Gagne R M 1975 Essentials of learning for instruction (expanded edn). The Dryden Press, Hinsdale, Illinois

Honey P, Mumford A 1986 The manual of learning styles. Printique, London

Hulse S F 1992 Learning theories: something for everyone. Radiologic Technology 63(3): 198–202

Jobling M H 1987 Cognitive styles: some implications for teaching and learning. Physiotherapy 73(7): 335–338

Knowles M 1983 The modern practice of adult education: from pedagogy to androgogy. In: Tight M (ed) Adult learning and education. Crook Helm in association with the Open University, London, ch 2, p 53–70

Marton F , Saljo R 1976 On qualitative differences in learning; outcome and process. British Journal of Educational Psychology 46: 4–11

Maslow A H 1943 A theory of human motivation. Psychology Review 50: 370–396

Mast M E, Van Atta M J 1986 Applying adult learning principles in instructional module design. Nurse Educator 11(1): 35–39

Neame R B L , Powis D A 1981 Towards independent learning: curricular design for assisting students to learn how to learn. Journal of Medical Education 56: 886–893

Piaget J , Inhelder B 1958 The growth of logical thinking from childhood to adolescence. Routledge, London

Rogers C 1983 Freedom to learn for the 80's. Charles E Merrill Publishing Company, London

Skinner B F 1953 Science and human behaviour. Macmillan, New York

Slevin O D'A, Lavery M A 1991 Self-directed learning and student supervision. Nurse Education Today 11: 368–377

Stengelhofen J 1993 Teaching students in clinical settings. Chapman and Hall, London p 55–57

Titchen A 1987 Continuing education: a study of physiotherapists' attitudes. Physiotherapy 73(3): 121–124

5 Factors influencing learning

Introduction

Theories on adult learning were reviewed in Section 4. There are, however, many other variables which can influence the quality and outcome of learning. These will be addressed in this section.

Aim

The aim of this section is to make you aware of the extent and diversity of the factors which may influence learning, and to demonstrate how to draw upon these factors when helping others to learn.

Objectives

By the end of this section you should be able to:

1. Identify factors which may influence learning.
2. Apply the factors under your control in a way which maximises learning.
3. Explain variations in level of performance.
4. Select appropriate learning methods.
5. Deliver feedback in a positive way.

An individual's ability to learn is not constant - anyone who has ever been a learner knows this. The capacity for learning depends upon a complex relationship, or transaction, between various factors.

ACTIVITY 5.1

Spend no more than 35 minutes on this activity.

1. Think back to a recent postgraduate course that you have attended. Write down a list of factors which might have had an impact on your ability to learn. Include in your list positive and negative responses.
2. A group of physiotherapy learners who had been out on clinical placement were asked to identify factors within these placements which had influenced their ability to learn. A list was then made from this feedback session, and is included in Appendix 1. You will notice that in this list there are both positive and negative factors.

Think back to your own experiences as a learner in a clinical setting. How would your list compare with that of these learners? Highlight any common factors.

Keep the lists for future use.

Most of the factors you have identified will probably relate to one or more of the following elements in some way:

- the learner
- the educator(s)
- the current learning context
- the learning environment
- the group of which the learner is a part.

All of these elements influence learning in some way, either positively or negatively. We will now consider each of them in turn.

The learner

In a previous section groups of learners were identified for whom a health professional might act as an educator. You will have noticed that individuals learn at different speeds and with varying degrees of understanding. A wide variety of factors will influence the individual's ability to learn. Within the same learner group the abilities of individual learners will vary according to age, maturity, past experience, stage of education, level of intelligence, motivation, enthusiasm, psychological state, attention span and other personality factors. Points that are important in relation to these areas are outlined below.

Age/maturity

These two factors are inextricably linked, although maturity of attitude, behaviour and thought is probably more important than chronological age. We all know of people who at 18 have the maturity usually associated with someone in their mid-forties and vice versa. A mature approach to the learning process is normally associated with positive outcomes, high levels of motivation and well-developed interpersonal skills. As a clinical educator you should be aware that the learner exhibiting mature interpersonal skills may mask gaps in knowledge and technical abilities, and that whilst interpersonal skills are vital in most healthcare settings they cannot stand alone. It is also important to recognize that the more mature learner is likely to be subject to potential additional pressures. These pressures are likely to be both external – e.g. their family situation, travel difficulties, financial problems and so on – and internal, i.e. they are generally driven by a greater need to achieve than are younger learners (pressures such as these should be remembered when considering psycho-social issues in Section 6).

It is possible that you will find yourself supervising learners who are older than you. The possibility for tension exists on both sides, and responsibility for managing the situation should be shared equally. You may well feel threatened by someone who is perceived to have greater life experiences, or who may be more highly qualified in another academic area. By the same token, a learner can easily feel demeaned by an educator who does not appear to recognise their worth. Both of these responses are likely to be an overreaction to the situation, and you should feel confident that as long as your knowledge and skills are at an appropriate level, you have nothing to fear. The more mature learner may ask highly challenging questions. In response you should not underestimate the breadth and depth of your own knowledge and clinical abilities, but at the same time you should be prepared to accept that you cannot know everything. In this situation, do not be afraid to admit what you don't know, but be sure to direct the learner to an appropriate source for that information. Equally, the learner (of any age) would be well advised that to test their educators with impossible questions or difficult attitudes is likely to have a negative effect on the learner-clinical educator relationship and hence on the learning process. Both parties have a responsibility to manage the learning process in a way that optimises the outcome.

Past experience

The past experience of learners will take many forms and may influence learning in a variety of ways. Some learners will have a headstart in relating to patients and colleagues by virtue of their previous employment and pastimes. This leaves them more able to concentrate on the areas of skill development and acquisition and application of relevant knowledge. Others may arrive in your workplace on the crest of a wave, having received glowing reports and high marks on a previous clinical education placement. Conversely, a poor or failed placement may have shattered the learner's confidence. In both cases there will be some effect on their expectations at the outset of the new placement and on their subsequent performance.

It is unlikely that you will be aware of either of these extremes unless the learner volunteers the information. It is important that if this is the case you do not allow it to influence your attitude towards the learner. Each placement is unique in the challenges it presents and in the skills and knowledge that it demands. In addition, the personal and social circumstances at the time of each individual learning experience can have a dramatic effect on performance.

Stage of education

The learner will arrive with knowledge and attitudes which are related to experience obtained prior to beginning the current educational programme. In addition, on professional courses learners will be placed with you at various stages in their professional development. This inevitably results in variations in learners' abilities to learn and in their performance, depending upon the exact nature of the previous experiences. Even where a supposedly similar pattern of experiences is planned for a number of learners, the precise nature of these will vary. For example, learners may go through a sequence of similar placements in terms of speciality and yet may have vastly different experiences.

ACTIVITY 5.2

Can you suggest possible reasons for there being discrepancies in experience between sequences of apparently similar clinical education placements?

Motivation

This is absolutely central to the success of any educational process. Unless the learner is motivated they are extremely unlikely to fulfil their potential regardless of innate ability. You can probably relate this to your own past learning and that of others you know well. Motivation may be defined as the desire to learn.

ACTIVITY 5.3

Consider for a few minutes the factors influencing your own motivation to use this package.

The points on your list may include extrinsic factors such as additional financial renumeration or the prospect of future promotion, and intrinsic factors such as increasing professional competence which would improve your own self-esteem. From the learner's perspective, the former may have to do with passing exams and assessments, achieving a high degree classification, qualifying for a profession and pleasing the educators. Intrinsic factors may have to do with satisfaction at success in a series of personal and intellectual challenges or with the desire to contribute to the care of people who are injured, disabled or ill.

External motivation is often transient in nature and ultimately gives less satisfaction than the achievement of personal goals of a more intrinsic nature. As an educator you should try to encourage the development of intrinsic motivation in your learners. This may seem an impossible task but you are likely to serve as a role model for many of the learners who work with you. As such, your attitudes towards your patients/clients and your profession, coupled with your enthusiasm, will influence their level of motivation. In turn this will be central to the learning process. It was mentioned earlier that pleasing the educator was an important extrinsic factor in motivation. On the face of it, it sounds unlikely, to say the least, that today's school-leavers, or the mature learners who will form their peer group, would be affected in this way. However, your interactions on a one-to-one basis may well result in a level of respect for you which will fuel the learner's desire to impress or please.

Your handling of the interaction between the learner and yourself is also crucial in terms of motivation, and central to this will be how you handle the task of giving feedback.

ACTIVITY 5.4

It would be useful for you now to reflect on your own experiences of receiving feedback and to evaluate the success of this process. Identify two or three approaches which aided your development and two or three that you can remember as hindering development or as being demotivating.

Thompson (1994) suggested that the educator should approach the business of giving feedback as follows:

- always begin with things that have been done well
- avoid reprimanding the learner with anyone else around
- call errors 'points to consider'
- set two or three goals (don't overwhelm the learner with problems)
- offer the learner your time
- admit when you don't know
- observe the learner sensitively in terms of their verbal/non-verbal messages.

Feedback content and style of delivery are vital to the task of motivating the learner and we will return to this subject in Section 7.

The topic of motivation would be incomplete without reference to Maslow (1943) and his theories concerning human needs. He identified five levels, or classes, of need arranged here in hierarchical order:

- self-actualisation
- self-esteem
- belonging
- health and safety
- physiological.

Each class of need is stronger than the one above it in the hierarchy, and when both are lacking the lower one is the more powerful in terms of motivation. For example, physiological needs are the most basic (hunger, thirst, etc.) and must be satisfied before the individual can attend to other needs at a higher level. Safety comes next and encompasses the need for security, stability and protection. Belonging involves friendship, affection and love needs. Esteem is concerned with achievement, mastery and competence, and self-actualisation, the highest class, is concerned with the fulfilment of personal potential.

This theory has obvious implications for anyone involved in any area of education. Whilst it may be impossible to ensure that the lower building blocks of the hierarchy are in place when helping others to learn, the theory may on occasion help to explain unexpectedly poor performance. Whether dealing with a learner health professional, a junior member of staff or a child undergoing postural re-education, their needs as learners are likely to differ considerably within the frameworks described above.

Level of intelligence

Intelligence may be considered as that which is measured by intelligence tests. It is a somewhat obscure concept. The argument about the relative influences of nature and nurture persists and some educators maintain that given the appropriate learning experience, 'all or almost all learners can master what they are taught' (Block 1971).

The institution's admissions process should have ensured that this is the position in which your learners find themselves. However, Block's theory does not specify time limits, and the constraints imposed by the curriculum of study will prevent the majority of learners from achieving mastery in the time available. Competence is a different matter but mastery may need to be postponed until the post-registration stage.

It is evident that many factors influence the learner's ability to learn. All these factors interact and are reflected in the level of performance. Some factors cannot be influenced by the educator but motivation is the most obvious exception. This should not be viewed in isolation but should be set alongside preparation, implementation of the learning experience and your manipulation of the learning environment.

The educator

As has already been seen, the educator plays a prime role in influencing the learning process. We now need to look at how the educator can help to optimise the learner's potential. The most successful clinical educators are those who are able to identify and respond to the individual learner's needs, thus facilitating their learning.

As was discussed in Section 2, the major responsibilities of the educator are to:

1. identify the learner's needs in conjunction with the learner
2. set clear, achievable and measurable learning objectives in conjunction with the learner and their institution
3. plan an appropriate programme which will act as a framework in which these learning objectives can be achieved, again in conjunction with the learner
4. facilitate the learning process as appropriate
5. appraise the learning that is taking place
6. identify/diagnose faults in the learning process
7. give appropriate feedback to the learner
8. manage change in the learning direction, if necessary

9. assess learning and give feedback to the learner

10. evaluate the quality of the learning experience.

You will review these responsibilities in Section 11.

Many educators are now formalising the stages in the above process by way of learning contracts. A learning contract has been defined by Berte (1975) as 'a written or verbal agreement or commitment reached between the parties involved in an educational setting regarding the particular amount of learner work or learning'. At a most basic level it identifies what a learner wants to learn, how they will go about learning it, how and by whom they will be assessed, and by what standards of performance they will be judged. See Section 7 for more information on learning contracts.

The relationship between facilitating and learning is very strong – the performance of the educator can influence the fulfilment of the learner's needs, and can have a major effect on the learning process.

Factors which influence the effectiveness of the educator are their:

- interpersonal skills
- motivation
- level of expertise
- security in their own role
- prior experience as an educator and learner.

All these points will affect the interaction between the educator and the learner, and also the educator's ability to motivate the learner. Vaughan (1994) suggests that the educator can maximise their effect as a motivator by:

- providing psychological support and making learning 'comfortable'
- providing feedback on progress
- being a suitable role model for learners to strive to emulate
- providing challenges for the learners, matched to ability, to stimulate them and further their development.

Under the section on motivation the needs of learners identified by Maslow (1943) were seen as being essential to the learning process. However, it is easy to forget that educators also have needs, and these must be taken into account in any successful learning experience. Sometimes, learners are so focused and anxious about their own requirements that they appear to be unaware of the educator's needs. This one-sided approach can lead to tensions which can compromise the educator/ learner relationship and ultimately the learning process. Some responsibility for fulfilling an educator's needs must also rest with the clinical manager, in terms of the level of support offered to clinical staff and the value attached to their work.

ACTIVITY 5.5

Now read Ramsden & Dervitz (1972) (see Reader, p. 55) who have addressed many of these issues. You will find much of relevance to current clinical practice.

The learning environment

The learning environment consists of several interrelated factors which can be summarized as follows:

1. physical environment

2. psycho-social influences
3. political climate
4. institutional/departmental structure, culture and ethos.

All these factors will be addressed in detail in Section 6.

The current learning context

Within the context of health professional educational programmes and linked clinical practice, the subject matter can be said to include:

● theory
● practical skills
● appropriate attitudes (influenced by values and beliefs).

In the clinical environment the learner faces the complex integration of all these elements. Their successful combination constitutes what Caney (1983) identified as professionalism. The difficulties associated with managing this interaction should not be underestimated by the educator or the learner. It is important to remember that it is very rare for learners to exhibit mastery of all three of the above elements sometimes known as learning domains (Bloom 1956). Furthermore, the extent to which these areas are developed will vary according to the area of speciality to which the learner is attached and the learner's stage of education.

Learners will enter the particular clinical setting with various levels of ability in the three learning domains. As an educator, you should be aware that the development and consolidation of these abilities will be influenced by, among other things, interpersonal relationships between the learner and the client, and the learner and the multidisciplinary team. In addition, the learner's personal and social circumstances will also have an impact. For example, students who are unhappy in their temporary accommodation and who are feeling remote from their friends and family may find it more difficult to learn.

Learners in groups

It is likely that on a day-to-day basis in the clinical setting most of your contact with learners will be one to one or within small groups. It is important, therefore, that you should focus on the strategies that are most relevant to these situations. In any group learning situation, the personalities of all members (learners and educators) will create specific group dynamics which will be of prime importance in shaping the learning experience. The personalities of the strongest and most influential members of the group will often have a profound effect on the group's character.

Techniques for enhancing group work draw upon the same fundamental principles and concepts of learning as those used in one-to-one situations. However, the actual techniques employed will inevitably differ. For example, it is important to draw upon the opportunities that are presented by virtue of the size of the group in order to make learning an active process which is pertinent, enjoyable and productive. Habeshaw (1988) and Gibbs et al (1984) suggest a variety of ways to facilitate learning in groups. Habeshaw deals with ways of making the most of the lecture setting, while Gibbs presents ideas for use with smaller groups. It is important that you select methods which are appropriate to the group size, constitution and subject matter. When both the subject matter and the group seem to warrant a formal presentation style you will need to plan the session carefully in advance, giving consideration to:

- aims and objectives
- content
- variation of style
- visual aids
- verbal delivery
- handouts
- room layout
- evaluation forms – if appropriate.

Where professional courses have a significant proportion of mature learners, some educators report that in general this has had a positive effect on the group. The maturity and life experiences of these learners will often inject a certain motivation and commitment into the group which has a beneficial effect on the learning process.

When you are involved in educating two or more learners at the same time, the opportunity exists for peer learning. This is where learners are encouraged to draw on each other's skills and knowledge, and also to collaborate in their work. Lincoln & McAllister (1993) explored the role of peer learning in clinical education and concluded that it was particularly beneficial for mature learners.

ACTIVITY 5.6

Read the Lincoln & McAllister (1993) article (see Reader, p. 61).

Could this approach be adapted for use within your service?

Have you been involved in this sort of approach as a learner? If so, what problems/benefits did you come across?

Summary

In this section, we have considered a range of factors that can influence the learning process. This should help you to understand variations in the performances of learners. It should also help in developing strategies to maximise the potential for learning.

REFERENCES

Berte N R 1975 Individualising education through contract learning. University of Alabama Press, Alabama

Block J H 1971 Introduction to mastery learning: theory and practice. In: Block J H (ed.) Mastery learning: theory and practice. Holt, Rhinehart & Winston, New York, ch 1

Bloom B 1956 Taxonomy of educational objectives: the classification of educational goals. Handbook 1 – Cognitive domain. McKay, New York

Caney D 1983 Competence – can it be assessed? Physiotherapy 69(8): 302–304

Gibbs G, Habeshaw S, Habeshaw H T 1984 53 interesting things to do in your lectures. Bristol Technical and Educational Services Ltd, Bristol

Habeshaw S 1988 53 interesting things to do in seminars and tutorials. Bristol Technical And Educational Services Ltd, Bristol

Lincoln M, McAllister L 1993 Peer learning in clinical education. Medical Teacher 15(1): 17–25

Maslow A 1943 A Theory Of Human Motivation. Psychology Review 50: 370–396

Ramsden E L, Dervitz H L 1972 Clinical education: interpersonal foundations. Physical Therapy 52(10): 1060–1066

Thomson S 1994 The nature of teaching and learning. In: Hinchcliff S (ed) The practitioner as teacher. Scutari Press, London

Vaughan J 1994 Assessing learning needs. In: Hinchcliff S (ed) The practitioner as teacher. Scutari Press, London

6

The learning environment

Introduction

As discussed in Section 5, the learning process involves a complex relationship between a number of variables. A key component of this process is the learning environment. It follows, then, that every endeavour should be made to create a favourable learning environment for each individual learner group.

Aim

The aim of this section is to help you to create a learning environment which is suitable for the needs of your learners.

Objectives

By the end of this section you should be able to:

1. Identify the major factors influencing the learning environment, with particular reference to those affecting the clinical learning environment.
2. Create a favourable environment for your learners.

Understanding the nature of the learning environment

The learning environment may be defined as:

A setting where educational opportunities are provided and maximized.
(Simms et al 1990)

An effective learning environment enables the learner to feel secure, encourages an exchange of ideas between the educator and the learner, values the learner's contribution to the learning process and promotes a sensitive approach by the educator.

Studies by Simms et al (1990) and Lickman et al (1993) describe the learning environment as a catalyst which governs the learner's enthusiasm, commitment and receptiveness to the learning process. These studies illustrate the power of the environment and the enormity of its impact, which must not be underestimated.

To enable you to appreciate fully its contribution to the learning process and to help you tailor it to meet the needs of your learners, we will now consider the interrelated factors that may have an impact on it. These factors, which were summarised in Section 5, are highlighted here in Figure 6.1 and will be expanded upon in this section.

Let us now consider each of these factors in turn.

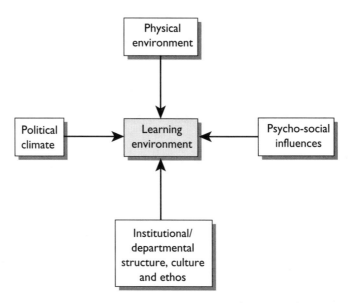

Figure 6.1 Factors comprising and impacting on the learning environment

The physical environment

When choosing the physical environment for learning, the college-based educator considers the category of learner, the number in the group and the learning objectives. Possible settings will include the lecture room, the library and the laboratory. In the clinical setting the educator may not have this choice, and settings will include wards, seminar rooms, patients' homes and clinics. You can probably add to this list.

Different teaching methods will be appropriate for different settings. There are many elements which constitute the physical learning environment. They include temperature, lighting, acoustics or noise level, and the atmosphere of the setting (e.g. is it non-threatening?) A small private area can often appear less threatening to the learner than a large, more exposed area.

Maslow (1954), who has already been referred to in Section 5, stressed the importance of meeting the basic physiological and safety needs of the learners before the higher intellectual needs can be fulfilled. Although this model may have been superseded by more recent ones, it continues to provide a useful framework for considering the needs of learners. The Chartered Society of Physiotherapy's 'Standards for clinical education' (CSP 1991) also recognises the need to meet these basic requirements prior to and during each clinical placement. 'Standard 5' requires that, in the placement area, the learner should be provided with information relating to changing facilities, canteen facilities, health and safety policies, etc. These requirements are considered to be imperative for the smooth running of any clinical education programme.

Shailer (1990) recognised the importance of the physical environment when setting criteria for audit purposes. She indicated the need for a private area where confidential feedback/discussion between the educator and the learner can take place. The value of such feedback and its contribution to the learning process has already been referred to in Section 5 and will be discussed in more detail in Section 7.

The requirements mentioned above can generally be met, but other physical influences, which have an equal impact on the environment, are more difficult to control.

You will be aware of recent social policy changes which have directed care away from institutions towards community settings. The advent of an increase in community-based practice has brought with it further challenges to both the learner and the educator. Unpredictable physical factors may be present. For example, in a patient's home, cramped living conditions or anxious relatives may alter the balance within the environment and impose additional stress on the learner. However, the positive aspects of a diverse environment must not be disregarded. Barris et al (1985) stressed that 'the objects, people and situations in the environment stimulate a person's interest and provide opportunity for action and consequently for development and maturation'.

In a comprehensive ethnographic study of the community learning environment, Mackenzie (1992) addressed issues concerning the learning process and the learners' experiences of learning within this diverse setting.

ACTIVITY 6.1

Now read the Mackenzie (1992) article (see Reader, p. 70). It will help you to appreciate the difficulties experienced by learners within the community setting.

How far can the learning environment be controlled by the educator?

The learning environment of the clinical setting has a unique and dynamic nature which at times can appear 'ungovernable'. In Ramsden & Dervitz's (1972) study, which you looked at in Section 5, you may have noticed that they identified factors which were outside the immediate control of those involved in the learning process, i.e. the clinical educator and the learner – 'These factors derive from the clinical setting itself.' This aspect of the clinical setting is influenced by a number of factors:

- the diversity of the clinical settings in which learning occurs
- the opportunistic nature of the learning experience within the clinical setting
- the spontaneous nature of the learning experience within the clinical setting
- the additional responsibilities of the clinical educator.

Mackenzie (1992) suggested that learners whose learning experiences 'straddle' both college- and clinically based settings may be more acutely aware of the diversity of influences on the learning environment than the educator.

To understand fully the impact of this dynamic clinical setting, it may be useful to identify the differences between college- and clinically based learning environments (see Table 6.1).

Table 6.1 A broad comparison of college-based and clinically based learning environments

College setting	Clinical setting
Learner and teacher are working together in a classroom. The focus of their activity is the current student learning objectives Learning needs are priority	Learner and clinical educator are working together, and with the patient. The focus of their activity is the patient's needs Patient's and learner's needs alternate as a priority The clinical education setting is dynamic
The environment should be relatively 'stable' A lecturer/tutorial/seminar/laboratory session can be prepared in advance and is therefore within the educator's control	Although detailed planning is and important part of the clinical education process, teaching and learning often occurs spontaneously in response to dynamic treatment situations. The clinical educator has less control

ACTIVITY 6.2

This activity should take you no longer than 30 minutes.

Enlist the help of a small group of colleagues, write down and discuss spontaneous ideas in response to the following.

Focus on a local clinical environment and a college-based environment with which you are currently familiar. Highlight any local and specific differences which may exist between these two environments. Discuss how these differences might impact on the learning experience.

Psycho-social influences impacting on the clinical environment

Psycho-social influences can be defined as the influence of social factors on human interactive behaviour. The quality of the relationship between the educator and the learner is the cornerstone on which all other factors affecting the learning environment rest.

Griffiths (1987) advocated the need to encourage an awareness of this interaction between educator and learner in order continually to appraise the environment and to maximise its potential. Ramsden & Dervitz (1972) highlighted the importance of the clinical educator gaining an understanding of the 'interpersonal bases of the learning experience'. Without this understanding, it is difficult for the educator to create an environment which is conducive to learning. Following a later study by French & Neville (1991), which examined the constituents of a 'good' or 'poor' clinical experience, clinical educators were encouraged to foster an environment which is 'collaborative and mutually respectful' while discouraging one which is 'autocratic and formal'.

ACTIVITY 6.3

Now read the whole of the Neville & French (1991) article (see Reader, p. 80). Think about the consideration of the impact of psycho-social factors on the learning environment.

The study by Emery (1984) which you looked at in Section 2 investigated both learners' and educators' perceptions of clinical education. Jarski et al (1990) carried out a similar study to identify those teaching behaviours which were thought to be most helpful in contributing to a positive learning environment, and to rank them alongside teaching behaviours which were found to be detrimental to the creation of a positive learning environment.

ACTIVITY 6.4

Below is a list of teaching behaviours identified as most hindering to the learning process.

The educator:

- questions learners in an intimidating manner
- corrects learners' errors in front of patients
- bases judgments of learners on indirect evidence
- fails to adhere to teaching schedule
- fails to recognise extra effort
- discusses medical cases in front of patients
- is difficult to summon for consultation after hours
- appears to discourage learner/faculty (staff) relationships outside of clinical areas
- gives general answers to specific questions
- fails to set time limits for teaching activities.

Rate your level of agreement with each of the above perceptions, e.g. strongly agree, agree, strongly disagree.

Ask a junior colleague to rank the importance of each perception from the learner's perspective.

Now read the Jarski et al (1990) article, which you will find in the Reader (p. 84).

Learner feedback as further evidence of the importance of the interpersonal relationship between the clinical educator and the learner

The following clinical placement evaluation was received from a junior learner on a BSc (Hons) degree course in physiotherapy. It further illustrates the importance of the interpersonal relationship between the clinical educator and the learner. Two clinical educators' approaches are described, which result in the same learner having first a negative and then a positive learning experience.

> 'The criticism received from the clinical educator, intended to be constructive, often had the opposite effect. It was sometimes delivered abruptly, and instead of encouraging and giving me confidence, the clinical educator just made me feel that everything I did was totally wrong.'

> 'I immediately felt more welcome than on my last placement. I did not feel at any time threatened by the criticism offered. My clinical educator gave constructive advice and encouraged me a great deal. At the start of the placement, I was quite open and honest with my clinical educator and felt able to identify problem areas. My clinical educator actually listened to me and we were able to work together in improving my skills.'

There is a whole host of other factors over which the clinical educator may have little control, but an awareness of these variables will enhance the clinical educator's responsiveness to the learner's learning. These are discussed below.

Levels of anxiety

French et al (1994) stress how important it is for clinical educators to recognise the learner's 'level of anxiety' which, if it is too high, will result in an inability to learn. On the other hand, if the learner's anxiety level is too low, there is a simultaneous decrease in motivation and increased lethargic response. Coles & Grant (1985) state that 'even the biorhythms of those involved can affect the environment'. It is therefore helpful if the clinical educator is aware of any emotional difficulties which may affect the learner. A learning environment built upon mutual trust will enable the learner to share their concerns with the educator.

A series of coping workshops was designed by Cupit (1988) to enable the learner to adjust to the transition from a college base to clinical practice. It has been shown that this transition period generates stress in the learner. The workshops explored the following areas:

- the learner's negative and positive feelings about the forthcoming clinical experience
- the learner's expectations of the clinical educators
- the educator's expectations of the learners (student's perspective)
- a patient's possible expectations of the learner.

The workshops resulted in honest opinions being expressed and learning contracts being developed between the clinical educator and the learner (for further information on learning contracts and their uses, see Section 7).

ACTIVITY 6.5

Read the Cupit (1988) article (see Reader, p. 90) to gain a clearer understanding of the aims of the coping workshops.

It is assumed from this article that there is a period during which it is recognised that learners are in transition. This is not always the case. The second part of this activity should help you to apply Cupit's theory to the needs of your learners.

How could a similar coping strategy be developed in your clinical setting?

Political influences

The impact of political influences on the learning environment may be as a result of:

- Policy at central government level, e.g. issues related to funding and organisation of educational settings.
- Policies and financial constraints at local level, e.g. within the NHS trust or other organisation of which your clinical setting is a part.
- Changes within your immediate clinical setting, e.g. policy changes, fluctuation in staffing levels, reprofiling of your service, staff morale.

You can probably think of others to add to the list.

Institutional/departmental structure, culture and ethos

Institutional/departmental environments were the subject of an article by Parlett (1977). This influential paper enhanced understanding of the learning environment in academic departments. The findings of this study are highly relevant to the clinical setting.

Parlett suggested that the context or surroundings (what Parlett terms the 'learning milieu') in which teaching and learning occur have as much influence on the learning process as do the tutorials, lectures and other methods of teaching. Parlett also suggested that many people disregard the importance of these surroundings: 'While few would deny the importance of a supportive and stimulating working environment for both staff and learners little systematic attention is given to appraising it as such.'

ACTIVITY 6.6

We now suggest you read Parlett's (1977) article in full (see Reader, p. 95). It will help you to understand the complexity of factors which determine whether the climate is favourable to, and supportive of, learning.

ACTIVITY 6.7

This activity is designed to help you understand the issues that Parlett raises.

Identify a specific learning environment that you have experienced. Reflect on how it felt to be a learner in that environment. How pertinent to your past experience are the issues raised in Parlett's article?

Now that you have explored all the aspects of the learning environment, the following activity will help you to investigate the way you may shape and influence the learning environment.

ACTIVITY 6.8

Summary activity

Think of all the possible factors which you as an educator can influence in the clinical education setting. Highlight these factors on a flow chart.

During this last activity, you will probably have identified some of the factors shown in Figure 6.2. Consideration of the environmental factors over which you as a clinical educator have some control should enable you to make some advanced preparation for future clinical placements.

Summary

Having completed this section, you should now be more aware of the major factors influencing the clinical learning environment and those over which you as a clinical educator have some control. This should enable you to create a more favourable environment for future learners on clinical placement.

We now move on to Section 7, where we explore the key factors contributing to facilitation of the learning process and discuss some of the methods of facilitation that can be used in the clinical field.

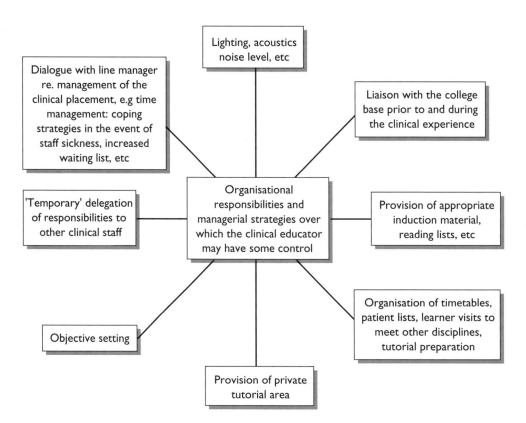

Figure 6.2 Factors over which the clinical educator has some control

REFERENCES

Barris R, Kielhofner G, Levine R E, Neville A M 1985 Occupation as interaction with the environment. In: Kielhofner G (ed) A model of human occupation: theory and application. Williams and Wilkins, Baltimore, p 42–62

Chartered Society of Physiotheraphy 1991 Standards for clinical education placement. CSP, London

Coles C R, Grant J 1985 Curriculum evaluation in medical and health care education. Medical Education 19: 405–422

Cupit R L 1988 Student stress: an approach to coping at the interface between preclinical and clinical education. The Australian Journal of Physiotherapy 34(4): 215–219

Dervitz H L, Ramsden E L 1972 Clinical education: interpersonal foundations. Physical Therapy 52(10): 1060–1066

Emery M 1984 Effectiveness of the clinical instructor: students' perspective. Physical Therapy 64: 1079–1083

French S, Neville S 1991 Clinical education: students' and clinical tutors' views. Physiotherapy 77(5): 351–354

French S 1994 Teaching and learning. A guide for therapists. Butterworth-Heinemann

Griffiths P 1987 Creating a learning environment. Physiotherapy 73(7): 328–331

Jarski R W, Kulig K, Olsen R E 1990 Clinical teaching in physical therapy: student and teacher perceptions. Physical Therapy 70(3): 173–178

Lickman P, Simms L, Greene C 1993 Learning environment: the catalyst for work excitement. The Journal of Continuing Education in Nursing 24(5): 211–216

Mackenzie A E 1992 Learning from the experience in the community: an ethnographic study of district nurse students. Journal of Advanced Nursing 17: 682–691

Maslow A 1954 Motivation and personality. Harper and Row, New York

Parlett M 1977 The department as a learning milieu. Studies in Higher Education 2(2): 173–181

Shailer B 1990 Clinical learning environment audit. Nurse Education Today 10: 220–227

Simms L M, Erbin-Roesemann M, Darga A, Coeling H 1990 Breaking the burnout barrier. Resurrecting the work excitement in nursing. Nursing Economics May-June: 177–187

7 Facilitating the learning

Introduction

Today's climate of ever-changing healthcare delivery is placing increasing demands on all healthcare professionals, including physiotherapists. It is therefore important, when facilitating learning, to acknowledge these demands and to encourage the individual learner to address such issues in their practice. In this way physiotherapists will be prepared to function efficiently in future healthcare environments. Practitioners of the future will need to be able to solve problems and set realistic goals, they will need a logical approach to the progression and termination of treatment, and they should be able, and motivated, to reflect on their own clinical practice.

Aim

The main aim of this section is to highlight the essential features of a successful facilitation process and to enable you to develop and use the skills that are required. The various methods of facilitation that are used in clinical settings will be presented and discussed.

Objectives

By the end of this section you should be able to:

1. Identify those who are involved in the facilitation process.
2. Identify the knowledge, skills and attitudes that need to be developed by the learner within the clinical setting.
3. Recognise the importance and use of feedback in the facilitation process.
4. Explore the methods of facilitation that can be implemented to enable the learner to achieve the placement objectives.

Let us first consider those who are involved in the process of facilitating learning.

Who can facilitate learning?

The clinical educator is generally the person who facilitates learning in the clinical field, but other members of the multidisciplinary team, and even the patient, may be involved in this process. In addition, the college link tutor may be asked by the clinical educator or learner to contribute by suggesting alternate methods of facilitation if the learning process is temporarily arrested, something that may occur if the learner is experiencing difficulties in achieving the placement objectives and is thus failing to progress.

What attributes do we need to encourage?

Before we explore the methods of facilitation let us consider what attributes need to be encouraged in the learner. The authors attempted to address this question in a recent clinical workshop that was designed for clinical educators who were about to receive students for the first time. The results of this workshop are highlighted in Box 7.1. The list is by no means a definitive one.

Box 7.1 Identifying the knowledge, skills and attitudes that need to be developed in a physiotherapist

Knowledge and intellectual ability
- intellectual ability
- theoretical knowledge
- critical thinking
- problem identification, analysis and solving skills
- reflective practice
- research awareness

Clinical skills
- clinical interviewing skills
- examination and assessment skills
- a reasoned approach to treatment progression
- ability to determine priority goals
- practical/therapeutic competence
- ability to monitor and evaluate treatment

Communication skills
- ability to communicate with patients, patient's relatives and colleagues
- ability to provide information and health education
- ability to negotiate and be assertive
- ability to teach and present information

Managerial skills
- ability to manage a workload
- ability to manage time efficiently
- ability to prioritise
- ability to take responsibility

Professional attitudes and awareness
- respect for clients' individuality, privacy and dignity
- ability to use initiative
- responsiveness to change
- willingness to learn
- self-directed learning approach
- awareness of current healthcare and professional issues

ACTIVITY 7.1

This activity should take you about 30 minutes.

Think about the opportunities to develop knowledge, skills and attitudes that could be offered in your own clinical setting.

Before we look at the various methods of enabling students to achieve their objectives in the clinical setting, we should look at the all-important partnership between the clinical educator and the learner. This partnership is one of the essential elements in achieving a positive learning experience. Any breakdown or failure to establish a viable working relationship will result in a poor-quality learning experience.

The clinical education partnership

The clinical education partnership is highly unique and is perhaps more private than that between college-based educators and learners. This is due to the nature of the clinical environment, where clinical educator and learner work in close proximity. The importance of both the educator and the learner contributing to this partnership was reinforced by Higgs (1992) who believes that, in the clinical setting, 'clinical educators as teachers, programme managers and role models, and students as self-directed learners, play critical roles in promoting learning'. The success of the partnership is enhanced by initial impressions, and many clinical areas have adopted a useful policy of sending letters of introduction to students prior to their clinical placement. These aim to 'break the ice' and they help to reassure the learner of both the clinical educator's and the department's commitment to their clinical experience. Failure of either party to demonstrate commitment has been shown to lead to a compromised learning environment and hence to a poor learning experience (Ramsden & Dervitz 1972; you will have read this article in Section 5).

The importance of this partnership, the values held by clinical educators and their attitudes towards their learners was also highlighted in a study by Kautzmann (1990). The main aim of this study was to identify the learning needs of clinical educators, by exploring their attitudes towards the principles of adult learning. Knowles's principles of adult learning (which you were introduced to in Section 4) were presented to the study participants in the form of a list of 13 appropriate values and attitudes. The participants were then asked to rank these in order of importance.

The following activity is designed to help you, as a clinical educator, to identify the values and attitudes that contribute to a sound working partnership between you and your learners.

ACTIVITY 7.2

This activity should take you about 40 minutes.

On completion of this activity, you should be able to recognise the importance of these values and attitudes in establishing a collaborative partnership between yourself and your learners. This should encourage you to adopt them in your day-to-day management of the clinical placement.

Rank the following attitudes, which have been adapted from Knowles's (1980) principles of adult learning (by Kautzmann 1990), in order of importance.

1. Respect for learner's feelings and ideas.
2. Learning to function as a team member.
3. Supervisor is a resource person and provides feedback.
4. Students deserve a thorough orientation.
5. Students can identify learning needs.
6. Importance of assessing student's knowledge at the start of fieldwork.
7. Collaborative development of learning objectives.
8. Importance of adjusting instruction to student's learning style.
9. Desirability of involving students in planning their learning.

10. Value of incorporating student's interests, skills and experience into the learning plan.
11. Ability to adapt teaching to student's level.
12. Collaborative development of evaluation criteria.
13. Involving students in evaluating their performance

Now read the Kautzmann (1990) article, which is in the Reader (p.104), and compare your rankings with the study findings.

Did you agree with the order of importance identified in the study?

Having considered those positive values and attitudes that enhance the partnership between the clinical educator and the learner, we will now identify some areas of conflict that may exist between them. Such conflict can detract from the strength of the partnership. It is therefore essential to explore coping strategies to deal with such situations.

Understanding the different roles and possible conflicts in the clinical education partnership

In addition to being clinical educators, senior clinicians have a number of other very different roles which may or may not impact on their teaching role. The following are examples of areas where possible conflicts may arise.

Patient primacy

Clinicians are required to balance the need to allow students to take some responsibility for their learning, by taking an active part in patient management, with their concern that patients should receive the best possible care. As senior clinicians they remain ultimately responsible for the provision of such care.

Students entering a clinical environment may need to be made aware of patient primacy. Students from higher education establishments are often more familiar with college-based environments, where students' needs are of prime consideration.

Management responsibilities

In the ever-changing healthcare climate, the managerial responsibilities of senior clinicians seem always to be expanding. The need to reduce waiting lists and to provide efficient and cost-effective patient care is ever present. While the clinical educator cannot include the learner fully in all managerial decisions, an awareness of some management issues may greatly contribute to the learner's professional development. Mature students may have had experience of other professional life and may therefore have something additional to contribute in this area.

Education of junior staff and provision of in-service training

Junior staff in rotational posts also require support and guidance from senior clinicians. It is therefore important for the clinical educator to balance the available time between students on placement and their junior colleagues on rotation. An imbalance in this area can be a further source of conflict. It may be possible to organise joint tutorial sessions. These may serve to enhance the juniors' professional development by encouraging them to work collaboratively with the learner in the planning of case presentations. It is also possible that junior staff will gain some satisfaction from guiding students.

Direct and indirect teaching styles

The clinical educator's direct and indirect teaching styles, along with differences between their own learning style and that of the learner, were identified in Section 4 as possible sources of conflict in this partnership. You may wish to refer back to this section to reconsider these issues.

Identification of the learning needs

The process of facilitation is enhanced if the clinical educator and the learner make time at the beginning of the clinical placement to identify the learner's needs and review the placement objectives. The needs of the individual learner will vary according to their past clinical experience, their year of study and their personal requirements. When assessing learning needs it is helpful if both the clinical educator and the learner consider the following:

- the knowledge, skills and attitudes that the learner already possesses
- appropriate strengths and weaknesses that have been identified during past clinical practice experiences
- what attributes the learner needs to develop
- what attributes the learner would like to develop.

Identification of the learner's needs helps to formulate the learner's own personal learning objectives, promotes active learning and may form part of a learning contract.

Key components of the facilitation process

The clinical educator should:

- provide a structured programme/timetable incorporating objectives that have been tailored to the learner's needs
- adapt their approach to the learner
- meet the needs of the individual learners
- provide observational and hands-on experience
- develop open communication channels with the learner
- promote active collaborative learning
- provide opportunities for the exchange of feedback
- provide the student with personal access at appropriate times.

In addition Stritter et al (1979) identified the following factors as being of vital importance in facilitating learning in the clinical setting:

- encouraging active participation
- positive attitude towards teaching on the part of the teachers
- emphasis on applied problem-solving rather than factual information
- student-centred instructional strategies
- humanistic orientation
- emphasis on reference and research.

It was stated above that the clinical educator and the learner may use a learning contract to formulate the learner's personal objectives, having initially identified their needs. Cupit (1988) suggested that a contract negotiated in the clinical setting greatly benefits the partnership between the clinical educator and the learner.

The Chartered Society of Physiotherapy's 'Standards for Clinical Education' document (1991) recommends that within the first week of the start of a clinical placement, a form of learning contract is agreed between the clinical educator and the learner. This may either take the form of a written document or be a less formal discussion. Learning contracts are becoming more widely used in the clinical setting. They are particularly useful in this context, as placement planning can be tailored to meet the needs of relatively small numbers and can be adapted within the confines of resource limitations (Higgs 1992).

Learning contracts

Over the last two decades there has been a change in higher education which has shifted the emphasis from teaching to learning and from the teacher to the learner.

Rogers (1969) dismissed teaching as 'a vastly overrated function' and felt that the underlying assumption, that 'what was taught was learned', was erroneous. Most educators now accept that force-feeding students is both ineffective and counterproductive. The heavy reliance on the lecture, together with the student passivity which that may entail, has been replaced in departments in many institutions by more student-centred approaches, the teacher becoming the facilitator of learning. One approach to facilitating learning which is now being widely used is the 'learning contract'. A learning contract was defined by Berte (1975) as:

> . . . a written or verbal agreement or commitment reached between the parties involved in an educational setting, regarding the particular amount of student work or learning, utilizing selected learning resources on the one hand, and the amount of institutional credit or reward for this work on the other, and recognising that the agreement can cover various lengths of time, any amount of work and all disciplines or areas of knowledge.

Knowles (1986) described learning contracts as 'an alternative way of structuring a learning experience, it replaces a content plan with a process plan.'

Some educators are unhappy about the legal connotations of the word 'contract'. Race (1992) preferred the word 'agreement'. His definition is 'an agreed action plan to achieve identified learning objectives and gain particular competencies, and provide suitable evidence of the development, where both sides retain the freedom to renegotiate the agreement in the light of developments.' Despite this, the term learning contract is widely found in the literature.

The main elements of a learning contract include 'the notion of active parties to the contract working in a collaborative relationship but with the responsibility for learning transferred to some extent to the student' (Paul & Shaw 1992). The format of a learning contract seems to be as variable as the settings within which it is used. At a most basic level it identifies what a student wants to learn, how they will go about learning it, how and by whom it will be assessed and by what standards performance will be judged.

Race (1992) gave a step by step approach which can be followed by the learner with assistance from a tutor:

- Work out what you need to learn or achieve.
- Turn your learning needs into targets (objectives, competencies to be gained).
- Plan how you will go about meeting those targets and what you will need to help you on your way.
- Work out exactly what you will be aiming to show as evidence that you have reached your target.
- Decide how your evidence should be validated – what standards are you aiming to match?
- Draft your proposal as the framework for an agreement, ready for negotiation.
- Negotiate your agreement with other people.
- Carry out the developments involved in your agreement.
- As and when needed, renegotiate the agreement in the light of how things are going.
- Reflect on your personal learning outcomes (over and above the reflection which may come from other people measuring your work).

Some undergraduate and post-registration courses are now based entirely on learning contracts. Many more use learning contracts for certain course elements. Learners embarking upon a course from a multiplicity of backgrounds and with vastly differing past experience may benefit from the individual approach of tailoring their pathway to their individual needs. Other benefits may include improvements in problem-solving, decision-making and time management and an increase in self-confidence. The flexibility of the learning process appeals particularly to those students who might be classed as 'independent learners'.

The limitations of learning contracts include the time-consuming nature of the process. Frequent one-to-one consultations are necessary during the development of the contract. Richardson (1987) recommended that there should be a maximum of 12 students to one teacher because of the increased workload. She contended that contract learning is therefore inappropriate for large groups. She also acknowledged that this style of learning may be difficult or inappropriate for some courses, especially those that have been particularly successful with a more traditional teaching role. Mazhindu (1990) identified a major drawback when statutory regulations for professional education demand that a course should be completed within a specified period of time. From the learners' perspective, those who prefer the traditional teacher-student role may be reluctant to accept the freedom to self-direct their learning. Several sources stress the importance of adequately preparing learners for the contracting process. This may include providing written resource material, articles on learning contracts, sessions on objective setting, group discussion and one-to-one consultation, and making sample contracts available. The contract may not be finalised until the student is several weeks into the course or clinical placement experience and further negotiation is likely to continue until close to the end of the placement. Race (1992) concluded by saying:

> 'Learning is done by people, not done to people [...]. The most important benefit of negotiable contracts is the increased sense of ownership that you can feel about the learning programmes you embark on, leading in turn to enhanced achievement.'

A definitive handbook (for use by physiotherapy students in the clinical field), which includes a sample learning contract, has been developed by Cross (1992). Details of the handbook are included in the list of resource material in Section 12.

The step by step approach to learning contracts stresses the need to renegotiate the agreement. Renegotiation will only be possible if some form of feedback is provided by both the learner and the educator.

Role of feedback in facilitating learning

Feedback should provide the learner with essential information about their current performance and professional progress. Unlike summative assessment and evaluation (which will be discussed in future sections), the provision of feedback should be an ongoing process throughout the learning experience. Feedback should elicit an appropriate response in the learner, enabling them to identify new goals and, with guidance from the clinical educator, to modify their performance to achieve those goals.

The value of feedback and its contribution to the learning process cannot be overemphasised. Students in both college-based and clinical settings derive great benefit from its regular and constructive use. This is particularly true in the clinical setting where the clinical educator provides feedback across the three major areas of clinical competence: knowledge, skills and attitudes. Through the appropriate and regular use of feedback, the learner is encouraged:

- to become more self-aware
- to explore their own knowledge and practice
- to develop towards professional competence

- to function more safely and effectively
- to reflect on their own practice.

These important issues are highlighted by Henry (1985), who introduced a model for using feedback to facilitate professional development.

ACTIVITY 7.3

Read the article by Henry (1985) (see Reader, p. 108). It will give you a full appreciation of how feedback can be used in the clinical setting to facilitate the learner's development.

Timing of feedback: when and where should it be given?

Feedback should be given at regular and appropriate intervals during the clinical placement period. Clinical educators may find it useful to include slots for feedback on the learner's timetable. This practice ensures that the importance of regular feedback is highlighted, thus avoiding its delivery on an ad hoc basis. Learners who reach the end of a clinical learning experience having received little or no feedback are often left feeling very frustrated. This problem is exacerbated if the final assessment by the clinical educator highlights areas of weakness of which the learner has previously been unaware.

Most physiotherapy courses use clinical assessment forms that include a halfway/interim report, which is completed by the clinical educator. This facilitates the feedback between the educator and the learner, and stresses the need for appropriate timing of such feedback. An example of a halfway/interim report is given in Figure 7.1.

Halfway/interim reports aim:

- to encourage the clinical educator to identify students' strengths and weaknesses
- to highlight areas where improvement can be made
- to agree the action necessary to ensure the objectives for the placement are met.

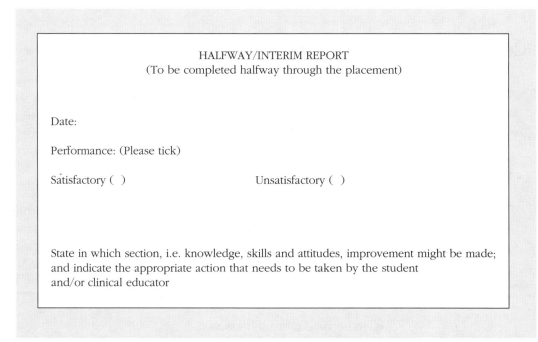

Figure 7.1 An example of a halfway/interim report for giving feedback

Goals set in response to feedback must be realistic, with both the clinical educator and the learner making collaborative efforts to achieve them. Feedback is usually verbal but, as mentioned above, an official form may be used. These are helpful in confirming:

1. that feedback has been exchanged
2. the nature of this feedback.

Such practice helps to avoid confusion and identifies learning needs. Stengelhoffen (1993) gives useful additional examples of forms used by different professional groups to record feedback sessions.

Who might contribute to the process?

In the clinical area, feedback is generally given by the clinical educator who is responsible for the day-to-day management of the placement. The visiting college tutor may contribute to the process if necessary and may be helpful in facilitating this exchange of information between the clinical educator and the learner. Finally, the role of the patient in providing feedback can be seen as an essential part of the learning process.

What form should the feedback take?

Feedback may be of a general nature, relating to the core placement objectives and the student's progress in the key areas of knowledge, skills and attitudes, or it may be of a more specific nature, pertaining to a particular skill. Feedback of a general nature is usually given at preset times during the placement, e.g. in the form of an interim/halfway report, but more specific feedback may need to be given on a more frequent basis, sometimes immediately after the event which provokes it, allowing the learner to adapt and develop their clinical practice. Feedback which aims to facilitate the learning process can take one of two forms:

- positive feedback
- constructive criticism.

Both types of feedback should aim to enhance the learning experience, but this is dependent on the method of delivery and on whether future learning needs are identified. A balance between positive feedback and constructive criticism must be achieved. Learners quickly feel demoralized if they are in receipt of only criticism, no matter how constructive, and confidence may be lost if no achievable goals are set or if sufficient guidance on how to achieve them is not given. It is also essential that, where possible, feedback is 'peppered' with positive comments and that a 'way forward' is agreed between the clinical educator and the learner.

ACTIVITY 7.4

This activity should take you about 40 minutes initially, with a further 30 minutes for discussion with a colleague.

Read the following scenario.

A second year physiotherapy student is on an outpatient placement for the first time. The student has reasonable interpersonal skills and is well motivated. However, the clinical educator feels that the student is not listening, either to them or to the patients. As a result of this inability to listen to essential information, the student is experiencing difficulty in accurately assessing the patients' needs and thus in providing an effective programme of care.

Reflect on the above scenario and then consider how you as an educator would attempt to address the problems experienced by this particular educator.

What additional resources would you consider accessing in an attempt to resolve the situation and to promote a positive learning outcome for the student?

Now list the possible approaches and methods of facilitation you could use.

If possible, ask a colleague who has had experience as a clinical educator to review your strategies. They may be able to come up with some additional solutions.

Methods of facilitation

One-to-one and small group teaching

Both one-to-one and small group teaching are used in the clinical field, but a high proportion of teaching is on a one-to-one basis. Clinical educators (who in addition to being responsible for facilitating learning also have their own caseload) often feel that the very essence of clinical practice is captured by 'on the spot' or 'on the hoof' teaching. This method has an inevitable spontaneity about it.

Initial observation of the educator by the learner

Learners working in a clinical area for the first time benefit from the opportunity of observing the clinical educator with a patient. This may involve the observation of:

- subjective and / or objective assessment procedures
- skill application and modification
- communication and collaborative goal-setting with patients, carers or other team members.

It is essential for the clinical educator to provide the learner with a structure for their observation, setting clear objectives for the observational period. This practice will prevent learners from becoming passive onlookers and will enable them to gain maximum benefit from this period. These objectives need to be identified in advance, thus allowing the learner to focus on a particular aspect of patient management and where possible to participate actively, i.e. to look, to feel, to listen and to discuss findings, as appropriate. Structured observation has been used successfully for many first-year physiotherapy students entering the clinical area for the first time. The assignment shown in Figure 7.2 is taken from a first-year student's workbook and forms part of their year 1 course assessment.

The extract in Figure 7.2 forms one of a series of assignments related to periods of structured observation in the clinical field. Subsequent assignments relate to the observation of:

- Manual handling skills – used in a clinical setting, with particular emphasis on environmental conditions.
- Departmental organisation – identifying the main responsibilities of an individual physiotherapist within a department.
- Communication skills – communication between a physiotherapist and patient, highlighting factors which enhance or detract from the therapeutic relationship.

These assignments form a useful resource tool for first-year students, they are used to develop initial reflection on practice and they may help to encourage the use of the 'professional practice diary', which will be referred to later in this section.

Observation of the learner by the educator

The need for the clinical educator to observe the learner irrespective of the learner's length of training may seem obvious but it is occasionally overlooked. Observation

ASSIGNMENT RELATED TO PATIENTS' PROBLEMS

Each of your visits provides an opportunity to observe patients with a wide variety of different problems.

a) For any two patients that you have observed during your visits, state what you considered to be their main *functional* problem, for each of these (problems) compile a list of:

1. the knowledge, e.g. anatomy of knee ligaments, that you might require to tackle the problem

2. the skills, e.g. how to measure a patient for a walking stick, that you might require to tackle the problem

Figure 7.2 An extract from a first-year student's clinical visit workbook

should be discreet and should be made at a distance. This practice allows the learner to maintain interaction with their patient and proves less stressful. Without appropriate observation and questioning at each stage of the learner's development, the clinical educator will be unable to make an accurate assessment of the learner's progress. Students left to their own devices, with no observation, will feel frustrated on discovering that a technique they have been performing for several weeks is both inaccurate and ineffective. This will result in a compromised learning outcome, and it raises obvious health and safety issues in relation to patient care.

The following quotation from a junior physiotherapy student working in an outpatient setting for the first time illustrates the frustration that learners can experience.

'I felt frustrated as I had been carrying out a technique on patients for the last week, only to discover when my educator watched me that I was doing it incorrectly. I was worried because I felt ineffective and may have damaged my patients.'

Through observing the learner's interaction with patients and questioning the learner after the interaction, the clinical educator can gauge the learner's readiness to progress and to take on more responsibility.

Scully & Shepard (1983) identified the 'diagnosis of readiness' as the first step towards moving the learner from initial observer to practising and competent clinician.

ACTIVITY 7.5

Now read the article by Scully & Shepard (1983) (see Reader, p.112). It will help you to appreciate fully the repertoire of 'flexible teaching tools' used by senior clinicians in their role as clinical educators.

Synonymous with the need to develop the competent clinician is the need to develop the autonomous or self-directed learner.

Development of autonomous or self-directed learning

This has already been discussed in Section 4. The constraints placed on this method of learning in the clinical field were highlighted, and are as follows:

- the need to adhere to professional core curricula
- time constraints
- ethical issues
- patient primacy

Clinical educators with experience of facilitating learning in the clinical field have developed innovative strategies for promoting self-directed learning, working within the boundaries of the above constraints. These strategies include:

- providing the learner with a contact list of multidisciplinary team members and allowing the learner to choose the team members they wish to contact during the placement period
- allowing the students to make their selection from a list of tutorials, case presentations, etc.

Both the above strategies, while encouraging self-direction, also serve to enhance the learner's skills in decision-making, time management, communication and prioritisation of their needs. Such strategies have obvious benefits for professional development.

Facilitation of the learner's knowledge base, skills and attitudes is also achieved by the following teaching methods which are particularly well suited to the clinical field. You will no doubt already be familiar with a number of these small group methods, which are often utilised during in-service training programmes. These methods can be readily modified and tailored to meet the learner's needs (French 1989).

Small group teaching

Small group teaching methods can be employed to promote the development of clinical skills and may include:

1. Role play with or without video feedback, for structuring and developing subjective and objective assessment skills. Role play is useful in the clinical setting but needs to be used judiciously and only by experienced people. If used effectively, it can promote skill development and facilitate the development of a problem-solving approach in the learner.
2. Tutorial sessions on specific skills, e.g.interpretation of chest radiographs, critical appraisal of journal articles, case presentations, etc.
3. Attendance by students of formal presentations, lectures, ward rounds or home visits.

Through the use of these various methods of facilitation, clinical educators are continually encouraging students to develop the knowledge base, skills and attitudes that are relevant to the clinical field in which they are learning, and to link this development with previous clinical experience. Higgs (1992) also advocates the use of small group teaching methods to facilitate the development of clinical reasoning skills in the learner, stressing the need to include adequate periods of time for the learner to reflect on practice. The need to promote the development of students as reflective practitioners is well recognised by the physiotherapy profession. In 1995, The Chartered Society of Physiotherapy relaunched its 'professional practice diary', which had been updated to accommodate the needs of undergraduates. This welcome adaptation ensures that students are now being encouraged to become reflective practitioners right from the start of their clinical practice experience.

Summary

> **Throughout this section, we have been identifying those involved in the process of facilitating learning in the clinical setting, and highlighting the key methods used to promote learning. The following article by Terry & Higgs (1993) encapsulates philosophies and strategies for the facilitation of learning which have been promoted in this section.**
>
> **SUMMARY ACTIVITY**
>
> Now read the article by Terry & Higgs (1993) (see Reader, p.122). It should stimulate you to reflect on your practice as a facilitator and enabler.

Now that you have worked through this section, you should be more familiar with the methods of facilitation used in the clinical setting. We move on now to Section 8, which addresses the purpose of assessment and explores the methods by which learners are assessed in both college-based and clinical settings.

REFERENCES

Berte N R 1975 Individualising education through contract learning. University of Alabama Press

Cross V 1992 Using learning contracts in clinical education. Queen Elizabeth School of Physiotherapy, Birmingham

Cupit R L 1989 Student stress: an approach to coping at the interface between preclinical and clinical education. The Australian Journal of Physiotherapy 34(4): 215–219

French S 1989 Teaching methods: student-centred learning. Physiotherapy 75(11): 678–680

Henry J N 1985 Using feedback and evaluation effectively in clinical supervision. Model for interaction characteristics and strategies. Physical Therapy 65(3): 354–357

Higgs J 1992 Developing clinical competencies. Physiotherapy 78(8): 575–581

Kautzmann L N 1990 Clinical teaching: fieldwork supervisors' attitudes and values. The American Journal of Occupational Therapy 44(9): 835–838

Knowles M S 1980 The theory and practice of adult education. Follett, Chicago

Knowles M S 1986 Using learning contracts. Jossey-Bass, San Francisco

Mazindhu G N 1990 Contract learning reconsidered: a critical examination of implications for application in nurse education. Journal of Advanced Nursing 15: 101–109

Paul V, Shaw M 1992 A practical guide to introducing contract learning. Learning contracts. Standing Conference on Educational Development (SCED), vol. 1, Paper no.71

Race P 1992 Not a learning contract. Standing Conference on Educational Development (SCED), vol. 1, Paper no.71

Ramsden E L, Dervitz H L 1972 Clinical education: interpersonal foundations. Physical Therapy 52(10): 1060–1066

Richardson S 1987 Implementing a learning contract. Journal of Advanced Nursing 12: 201–206

Rogers C R 1969 Freedom to learn. Merrill, Columbus, Ohio

Scully R M, Shepard K F 1983 Clinical teaching in physical therapy education. An Ethnographic Study. Physical Therapy 63(3): 349–358

Stengelhofen J 1993 Teaching students in clinical settings, 1st edn. Therapy in practice 37. Chapman and Hall, London

Stritter F, Hain J, Grimes D 1975 Clinical teaching reexamined. Journal of Medical Education 50: 876–882

Terry W, Higgs J 1993 Educational programme to develop clinical reasoning skills. Australian Physiotherapy 39(1): 47–51

The Chartered Society of Physiotherapy 1994 Professional practice diary, 2nd edn. Chartered Society of Physiotherapy, London

The Chartered Society of Physiotherapy 1991 Standards for clinical education placements. Chartered Society of Physiotherapy, London

8 Assessment

Introduction

There is often confusion between the terms 'assessment' and 'evaluation'. In this package, as in Rowntree (1987), 'assessment in education can be thought of occurring whenever one person, in some kind of interaction, direct or indirect, with another, is conscious of obtaining and interpreting information about the knowledge and understanding, or abilities and attitudes of that other person'. Evaluation is covered in depth in Section 9 and relates to the monitoring of the quality of an element of a course or a complete course. Assessment results will usually be part of the evidence gathered during the process of evaluation. Not all texts will use the terms in the same way, and you will find that some sources use 'evaluation' in the context of rating performance.

> *We spend our lives assessing others, trying to know them and explain them to ourselves – and often influencing them by our consequent decisions.* (Rowntree 1987)

In your everyday social interactions you will be aware of 'weighing up' other people – deciding whether you can trust them, whether you like them or whether you think they're good at their job. In parallel, you will be a target of their contemplations. More formally, you will have been assessed by doctors, teachers, driving test examiners and many others. Part of your role as a clinical educator, as you have already seen, is to take on the formal mantle of assessor.

This section first looks at some general issues and background relating to the assessment process, in particular the link between learning objectives and assessment criteria and their relationship to the assessment of competence to practise. It then goes on to look more specifically at what assessment is, what methods may be used, what is actually assessed, why assessment is carried out, who is involved in assessment, and how to assess.

Aim

The aim of this section is to enable you to contribute effectively towards the overall assessment of a student's competence while they are on clinical practice.

Objectives

By the end of this section you should be able to:

1. Explain what assessment is.
2. Discuss the purposes of assessment.
3. Distinguish between evaluation and assessment.

4. Identify areas of learning which may be assessed in the workplace.
5. Recognise different levels of learning within these areas as an aid to carrying out assessment.
6. Identify who carries out the assessment process.
7. Discuss behaviours which will facilitate or jeopardise the assessment process.
8. Describe different types of assessment and discuss their relevance to the clinical setting.
9. Recognise and discuss possible repercussions of inaccurate assessment.

The learner's perspective

You will be involved in assessing learners during their clinical education placements and you may also be asked to contribute to assessment at other times. During placements, major opportunities exist for the integration of theoretical knowledge, practical skills and interpersonal and intrapersonal abilities (self-awareness, self-control, self-confidence and the recognition of the impact of one's actions on others) and also for the assessment of these areas. The assessor needs to appreciate the difficulties the learner will have performing a balancing act that incorporates these three elements. For many students (and this is particularly true of recent school leavers), communicating effectively with the patient (and the educator) effectively in their new role will be enough of a challenge. To attempt, at the same time, to evaluate the patient's current status and make decisions about appropriate treatment techniques may seem awesome. Furthermore, to juggle these elements while trying to apply a technique requiring dexterity may sometimes seem impossible – and all this with the clinician (the expert) observing every move as part of continuous assessment. Amazingly, most students survive this sort of ordeal on a regular basis and come through relatively unscathed and with pass grades.

Learning objectives, assessment criteria and competence

As discussed in Section 2, it is usually the responsibility of the student's academic institution, in collaboration with senior clinicians, to identify core objectives for each placement speciality. Local objectives will be added to the list where a placement offers unique opportunities for learning. Both core and local objectives will probably be set some time prior to the student commencing a particular placement. At the beginning of the placement, the core and local objectives that have been set will be tailored to the needs of the individual student and may take the form of a learning contract or negotiated learning agreement, i.e. an agreement arranged between the student, clinician and visiting tutor. Learning contracts were considered in Section 7.

The learning objectives will relate to the development of competence, on which much has been written. Assessment of the learner on a vocational course, such as physiotherapy, will indicate whether the learner is competent (or otherwise) to practise. Competence has been defined as 'possession of the knowledge, skill and attitudes enabling an individual to perform fully in a basic professional role' (Higher and Further Education Working Party 1979). Caney (1983) suggested that it is reasonable that, at the point of qualification, competence should be assessed in terms of knowledge, skills and attitudes, but she feels that it is more than the sum of these three parts. She identified an acceptable speed of performance as one additional parameter. Competence to practise may be regarded as a phase in development preceded by incompetence and succeeded by proficiency and ultimately by mastery. The precise definition of these terms and the way in which they manifest themselves practically is open to debate, and the knowledge and experience of those involved in the process of assessment is crucial to maintaining appropriate standards. As a clinician involved in assessment, you should recognise that the competence you seek to help the student to achieve is only a stepping stone *en route* to mastery. While maintaining high professional standards, it is unrealistic to expect mastery in the time-scales available to the undergraduate.

The prime goal for all physiotherapy undergraduates is that they should reach the level of competence to practise. Core guidelines relating to the development and assessment of competence are set by the Chartered Society of Physiotherapy (CSP) (1991) and are reflected in the placement objectives and criteria for assessments set by individual schools of physiotherapy. Academic and clinical staff often have a gut feeling that someone is ready (or totally unsuitable) to qualify. Such subjectivity is not enough. Both academic and clinical tutors need to apply knowledge and experience to the consideration of criteria for competence in a way that gives reliable, valid and fair results.

ACTIVITY 8.1

Read the article by Caney (1983) (see Reader, p. 127). Decide if the article is relevant to current practice.

What is assessment?

When assessment takes place during a course of study and the student is able to benefit from feedback on their performance this is known as *formative* assessment. Strengths and weaknesses should be identified and discussed constructively and the student should be able to build on the feedback.

Summative assessment usually takes place at the end of a unit of learning and its purpose is to label or act as an indicator of achievement. It can take a number of forms but formal written and practical examinations are obvious examples, with all the accompanying stress, reliance on feats of memory and regurgitation of information.

Clinical assessment may well fulfil both roles (having formative and summative elements), but the continuous nature of the assessment process, usually over several weeks, may well remove some of the less desirable elements of certain modes of summative assessment.

Methods of assessment

Since the move of physiotherapy courses to higher education and the instigation of internal methods of assessment, the styles of assessment have diversified.

The assessment of the student's performance during clinical placements may take a variety of forms:

- Continuous assessment throughout the placement based on set criteria and a rating scale. This is usually carried out using a standard form produced by the academic institution and may involve overall performance and/or the successful completion of particular techniques or tasks (see Appendix 2 for an example assessment form). The criteria may vary for different stages of experience or for different types of placement. This would very much depend upon the particular pattern of clinical placements and the constraints influencing the organisation of the clinical programme.

- Assessment using the negotiated criteria of the learning contract, in a manner agreed by those involved (this is covered in more detail in Section 7).
- A formal assessment in which the student demonstrates their ability to assess and treat a patient or perform a discrete practical task while being observed by a clinician and a visiting tutor (or some other combination).

Outside the clinical setting, assessment may take many forms, of which the following are only a few:

- written or practical examinations
- multiple choice questions
- essays
- seminar presentations
- projects or dissertations
- research critique.

These methods are outside the immediate scope of this package but you will find information on them in any standard educational text.

While examinations are usually formal, one-off, 'big bang' events, attempts are sometimes made to moderate the stress involved and to reduce the reliance on memory by adopting 'open book' or 'seen question' examinations. The formats of these types of examination are indicated by their names, and in both cases the learner can use books and articles to help them with their answers. The aim of such examinations will usually be to ascertain analytical and evaluative abilities rather than the ability to regurgitate facts.

The other methods of assessment in the above list may well be used as part of a 'continuous assessment' process, allowing the student to work at their own pace, in their chosen environment and making use of whatever learning resources are at their disposal.

There are advantages and disadvantages associated with any form of assessment, and certain types of assessment will be preferred by particular students. In attempting to be fair to students and also to produce realistic results with useful feedback, most courses will use a variety of methods and a number of staff in the assessment process.

What is assessed?

The learning objectives reflected in the assessment criteria must, at a minimum, relate to the core curriculum for each of the areas of clinical experience (Chartered Society of Physiotherapy 1991). Individual institutions will vary in the emphasis given to different areas of the curriculum. There will be many reasons for this, but staff expertise and local availability of particular specialists and placements will be major factors.

In reaching decisions about topics to be included in the assessment process, attention is paid to the relative importance of specific areas, and it is vital that the assessment criteria achieve a balance among the topic areas that 'must' be known, those that 'should' be known and those that it would be 'nice' to know. This should avoid the overemphasis of obscure areas yet help to distinguish the very able learner from the average.

In the stages leading up to a decision about whether the learner is competent to practise (and therefore to graduate), the development of knowledge, psycho-motor and interpersonal skills will be regularly monitored. Within these three areas there will be a wide range of ability, and the specific knowledge, skills and interpersonal behaviours required may well vary from one clinical speciality to another.

Box 8.1 The cognitive domain: a summary of educational objectives (Bloom 1956)

LEVELS

1. **Knowledge** by simple recall
   – of specific information
   – of ways and means of dealing with specifics
   – of generalisations, laws, abstractions
   e.g. to describe, to define, to list.

2. **Comprehension**
   – translation of information into a new form
   – interpretation of information
   – extrapolation from given information
   e.g. to interpret, to translate, to understand.

3. **Application**
   – of known ways of working in unfamiliar situations
   – of abstractions in particular situations
   e.g. to relate, to explain, to demonstrate.

4. **Analysis**
   – of the components of an argument, facts, theories; recognition of unstated assumptions
   – of relationships
   – of organisational principles
   e.g. to analyse, to identify.

5. **Synthesis**
   – combination of number of elements into coherent whole
   – production of a unique communication
   – production of a plan
   – derivation of a set of abstract relationships
   e.g. to formulate, to compose, to organise.

6. **Evaluation**
   – judgement by internal evidence
   – judgement by external criteria
   e.g. to assess, to evaluate, to compare and contrast.

It is an essential step in the development of a course or an element of a course that the required behaviours are identified in advance (objectives), that appropriate learning strategies are employed to encourage their development and that any assessment reflects the set learning objectives.

Taxonomies of educational objectives classify them into the three areas (or domains) previously identified (knowledge, psycho-motor and interpersonal skills). Within each category, different levels of learning are specified. Each successive level incorporates the levels below, thus forming a hierarchy (Bloom 1956, Krathwole 1964, Simpson 1972).

Each of the domains will be considered in turn, beginning with knowledge – the cognitive domain (see Box 8.1).

The cognitive domain

In formulating course objectives in the cognitive domain, educationalists will draw upon the principles demonstrated in Bloom's (1956) taxonomy. For an honours degree such as physiotherapy, a progression of level from year to year would be apparent and final-year objectives would draw largely upon the highest tiers (6 is the highest) of the hierarchy.

In attempting to assess students' abilities within the domains there will be certain types of assessment which are better suited than others to the domain in question.

ACTIVITY 8.2

This should take no longer than 20 minutes.

Can you identify assessment methods that could be used to assess the cognitive domain?

Check the clinical assessment criteria of a course with which you are involved. Do any of the criteria relate to the cognitive domain. If so, at what level?

In fact, the cognitive domain is probably the one which lends itself most readily to assessment by a wide variety of methods. This is particularly true of the lower levels.

The psycho-motor domain

A large percentage of the work of a physiotherapist can be classified as 'practical' and involves the acquisition of skills in psycho-motor tasks. Box 8.2 shows the stages involved in this process.

ACTIVITY 8.3

The psycho-motor area obviously applies to a wide range of everyday and professional tasks. Read the list in Box 8.2 again, but this time relate the levels to the process of learning to drive a car or the acquisition of skills pertinent to your own area of practice – perhaps the development of handling skills for the patient with neurological impairment or musculo-skeletal problems.

Suggest methods of assessment that are likely to be appropriate to activities within this domain.

Suggest methods of assessment which you feel may be inappropriate.

It is important to note that learners at undergraduate level may not reach the highest levels of this hierarchy in every (or any) area of skill development.

The affective domain

This domain relates to the development of values and attitudes. It has particular significance for the 'caring professions', and ability in this area is traditionally

Box 8.2 The psycho-motor domain: summary of educational objectives (Simpson 1972)

LEVELS

1. **Perceptual ability**
   – e.g. awareness through the senses.

2. **Readiness**
   – e.g. knowing what to do and how to do it.

3. **Learning parts of skill**
   – e.g. by imitation, practice.

4. **Habitualisation**
   – e.g. internalisation of a skill.

5. **Performing complex motor acts**
   – e.g. automatic performance of coordinated skill.

6. **Adapting and originating**
   – e.g. devising original ways to skill performance according to individual perception.

Box 8.3 The affective domain: summary of educational objectives (Krathwol et al 1964)

LEVELS

1. **Receiving** (attending)
   – awareness (conscious of what is happening)
   – willingness to receive (will tolerate what is happening)
   – controlled attention (will attend carefully to what is going on).

2. **Responding**
   – acquiescence in responding (learner reacts)
   – willingness to respond
   – satisfaction in response (sense of pleasure is evoked).

3. **Valuing**
   – acceptance of a value (it is seen to have worth)
   – preference for a value (sense of commitment)
   – commitment (high degree of certainty).

4. **Organisation**
   – conceptualisation of a value
   – organisation of a value system (an ordered set of relationships is beginning to occur).

5. **Characterisation**
   – beliefs, ideas and attitudes fused together in an overall view of life.

reflected in the interpersonal and intrapersonal (self-awareness etc.) skills of the learner (see Box 8.3).

The level attained by an individual in any particular area of behaviour will be reflected in their skill during interpersonal interactions. This is probably the most difficult area to assess. Direct observation is the most frequently used method, but it can lead to an undesirable amount of subjectivity unless criteria are tightly structured and the assessor has well-developed powers of observation and is self-aware.

Issues relating to the affective domain are usually assessed in clinical practice in relation to the learner's ease and appropriateness of interaction with patients, carers, staff and peers.

Having briefly considered the purposes of assessment at the beginning of this section, let us now consider why it is necessary.

Why assess?

Ideally, assessment and learning are closely bound together – the style of assessment should reflect the learning experience. The reasons for assessing are various and involve the learner, their host institution (university) and the profession to which they aspire.

ACTIVITY 8.4

This activity should take about 10 minutes.

Consider the reasons why assessment of the learner's ability during clinical education placements should be carried out. You may wish to think of these in terms of the benefits to the learner, the host institution and the profession.

List the reasons and then compare them with those identified below.

For the learner, good assessment should encourage and motivate both in anticipation of the event and by the feedback that is subsequently given. It should help to consolidate learning and, of course, provide a record of achievement to be used in the future; in addition, it should give some guidelines as to how performance might be improved.

For the host institution, assessment serves to monitor an individual student's performance as well as the overall success of a programme of study. The results will be used in combination with other assessment outcomes as 'evidence' to support the student's progression from year to year, and in combination with other elements ultimately to demonstrate their competence to practise. The student's host institution is likely to be the body awarding the academic qualification – the stamp of approval. In physiotherapy, automatic eligibility for state registration and membership of the professional body (which implies licence to practise) follows graduation from a course that is validated by the professional body.

In addition, assessment results will be used as an element of the evaluation process and therefore as part of the quality system for monitoring the success of a course.

The profession now delegates responsibilities of 'gatekeeper' to the institutions that are validated to provide physiotherapy education. However, there must be confidence that standards are being maintained and that the public can be assured of optimum levels of competence to practise. The Chartered Society of Physiotherapy and the Council for Professions Supplementary to Medicine monitor the quality of courses in the UK by representatives of the Joint Validation and Recognition panel (JV & R) attending joint validation events for new courses, by regular review of existing courses and by the external examiner system.

External examiners are appointed for each course from a list of senior educationalists compiled by the Chartered Society of Physiotherapy. Two or three external examiners will usually be involved with a course at any one time, and their involvement will usually be for a 3- or 4-year period. Their role is essentially twofold and is primarily concerned with fairness to students and with ensuring that standards are comparable with similar courses elsewhere. External examiners usually comment on the appropriateness of examination papers and other assessment methods prior to completion by the student. Subsequently, they sample a selection of marked work to check that grades have been allocated consistently and appropriately by the assessors. In addition, with practical courses such as physiotherapy, they may visit some clinical placements and discuss issues relating to the course with clinicians and students. When formal assessment events take place in the clinical setting, they may wish to observe the process at a location chosen at random.

Thus, the external examiners provide a dispassionate opinion on the quality and standards of set assessments and student performance. They attend end-of-session examination boards and assist the course team in making appropriate decisions about student progression. In addition their opinion is usually sought when minor changes to course structure are proposed. Major changes would have to go through appropriate committee (validation) channels within the host institution.

Who assesses?

In current practice in the UK, physiotherapy students are likely to undertake placements in a succession of different clinical units. The actual pattern of placements will vary widely depending upon numerous factors to do with the organisation of the curriculum and both physical and human resources. The clinical educators in each clinical placement must be experienced physiotherapists, showing a commitment to the education of students and to their own continuing professional development.

Over a sequence of clinical education placements the student might typically work with 6 to 12 clinicians. Each clinical educator will be using the same (or similar) guidelines or criteria in order to reach their conclusions about the student's abilities and potential. Safeguards have to be in place to ensure the reliability of marking. Clinical educators' courses and information days are very valuable in this process, and the criteria and rating scales are crucial.

While striving for objectivity in marking, it is inevitable that some subjectivity will creep in, due to the individual characteristics of the assessor and their past experience. This subjectivity may go beyond pure professional considerations. It is vital that as an assessor you recognise that your values, attitudes, beliefs and prejudices could have an impact on the marks you award to a particular learner.

In formal written examinations it is possible to make the assessment process anonymous, thus removing the positive or negative effects of discrimination. This is obviously not possible with practical assessment, but it is a major issue and recognition of your own values and attitudes may well be a vital step in ensuring fairness to students.

Some variability of marking between assessors is probably inevitable and this issue is likely to be addressed at course-specific information days run by individual schools and in regional clinical educators' courses, which usually cover general issues relating to the role of clinical educator. Certain safeguards exist: each assessor will be using the same criteria and rating scales to mark learners from the same establishment; several assessors will be involved in the overall process of clinical assessment, which will tend to moderate the effect of extreme marks when they are combined; some academic institutions may in addition use their own staff to collaborate with clinicians in reaching a representative mark.

The good assessor needs to have:

- *knowledge* of the subject area and the learning objectives
- well-developed clinical, interpersonal and communication *skills*
- appropriate *attitudes* with regard to the learner, sensitivity and empathy towards the patient/client, and professionalism in the role.
  (You may wish to refer back to the taxonomies relating to these areas.)

Ideally, the behaviours exhibited by the assessor will be similar to those expected of the clinical educator, as assessment is a central component of the educator's role. It is unlikely that the educator who is unapproachable, superior in attitude, uses sarcasm, criticises in front of others, concentrates on weaknesses and gives inadequate feedback will provide a good learning experience or help the student to maximise their potential in terms of assessed performance.

Traditionally in physiotherapy education, it has been the teacher or educator who has carried out the assessment. In the transition from the didactic role of the teacher to a predominantly facilitatory role, the emphasis has shifted from students passively receiving information to students taking responsibility for their own learning process. As part of this student-centred approach some institutions consider that students' participation in their own assessment is a natural development. Quinn (1995) points out that 'self-assessment seems to be one of the hallmarks of a professional practitioner in any field, so this is a practice that should be encouraged from the outset'. Self-assessment may fall short of student involvement in grading their own performance, and there are obvious potential problems. However, in most forms of assessment, the student should be involved actively during the feedback process in order to encourage reflection and self-evaluation during the review of various aspects of performance. Most students will tend to undervalue their performance, and some courses in some institutions will encourage negotiation between the educator and learner in reaching conclusions about grades. Where issues of professional competence are concerned, this process would have to be tightly organised and monitored. Boud (1995) considers issues relating to self-assessment at length.

As well as self-assessment, many institutions will include opportunities for peer assessment within their schedules. This may take the form of a discussion among small groups of learners, where comment and feedback on each other's performance is encouraged. Systems are sometimes devised on this basis so that a certain percentage of available marks may be allocated by the group. As with self-assessment approaches there are obvious possibilities for abuse but both methods are used widely and constructively.

How to assess

In the role of assessor, it is important for the clinician to be able to break down the complex tasks they observe and, by subsequent pertinent questioning, to differentiate the student who outwardly performs well (i.e. who has impressive interpersonal and practical skills) but has little in-depth knowledge from the learner who gives an equally impressive performance but also has a sound knowledge base to support any decisions about future progression or change in treatment. While well-developed interpersonal skills are of course essential, it is vital that they should not be permitted to mask shortcomings in knowledge, practical ability, decision-making and evaluation.

In any particular clinical setting the assessment criteria that need to be succesfully achieved are identified prior to the student beginning the placement; these must obviously relate directly to the syllabus and to the learning objectives.

The lists of criteria are usually linked to rating scales, which may be either numerical or alphabetical. The clinical educator has to draw on their own experience, knowledge base and practical expertise in reaching conclusions about the level of performance of any particular student for any particular task related to the set criteria. It is important that the clinical educator should set (and demonstrate) sufficiently high standards to ensure that the students ultimately gaining entry to the profession have achieved a level of competence to practise that will serve the needs of the patient and the service, and form a firm foundation on which to build to proficiency and ultimately mastery in a chosen speciality.

The use of lists of criteria and rating scales are widespread in physiotherapy education today but this was not always the case and several decades ago assessment of clinical practice was much less organised. An article by Forster & Galley (1978) was probably quite influential in this change. The rating scales used in conjunction with lists of criteria will usually provide between three and seven options to quantify the level of performance.

The assessor gathers information on the student's performance mainly through observation and by questioning/listening. The 'evidence' is gradually accumulated by continuous assessment.

ACTIVITY 8.5

Cross (1983) considered the use of rating scales and criteria at pre-registration level and with junior staff. Read the Cross (1983) article (see Reader, p. 130).

Some authors have reservations about criteria-based approaches to the assessment of competence. Girot (1993) reviewed the literature relating to the assessment of nurses' clinical practice and considered opinion relating to, for example, more intuitive approaches. Read the Girot (1993) article (see Reader, p. 135) and reflect on its content.

Observation

In order to observe in an effective way you need:

- To know what it is you are looking for.
  Consider, for example, a psycho-motor skill (such as a manipulation technique): you need to be able to break the task down into the component parts necessary for its effective and safe completion. Is the patient positioned correctly? Is the learner standing in an appropriate position? Has the exact anatomical area for treatment been localised? Is the technique applied correctly? All these points and more will have to be taken into consideration in deciding the level of performance demonstrated by the learner.
- To allow sufficient time to build up an accurate impression about the level of performance.
- To be aware of the possible impact on the learner of your presence and to try to minimise any adverse effects.

Questioning/ listening

Phrasing questions correctly is a skill to be learned:

- It is important that you should have an encouraging manner.
- Do not give the student the impression that you are trying to catch them out.
- The subject matter of the question should be relevant and should mainly fall into the 'must know' category.
- Ensure the wording is clear and concise and give the student feedback on their answer.
- A little gentle probing with questions beginning with 'why' will sometimes reveal gaps and misconceptions.
- Bear in mind the levels of the taxonomies and phrase questions appropriately for the level you expect from the learner. Questions purely aimed at facts (the lower levels of the hierarchy) will not be suitable for assessing the third-year student, who should be showing evidence of the evaluation and synthesis of information.

In order to gather convincing evidence, it is part of the educator's role to organise relevant learning and assessment opportunities; ideally, the two dimensions should occur in parallel. To do this effectively, the educator must have carefully considered the student's current level of knowledge and abilities and have identified gaps that need filling or areas in need of enhancement through experience.

On placements of several weeks duration, the gradual progress of the student is monitored and a steep learning curve should be expected. In trying to assess the level of performance, you need to allow sufficient time for observation, as mentioned above, and to look for some consistency at an appropriate standard. As

Stoker (1994) points out, once is an event, twice is a coincidence, but three times shows that there is a consistent pattern emerging.

Constructive feedback is absolutely essential and the student can make some errors *en route* without unduly jeopardising the final mark.

As we have seen, in physiotherapy clinical practice, performance is usually compared against standard criteria (criterion-referenced assessment). This form of assessment does not depend on comparison with others and is the basis of 'mastery' learning (Block 1971). In theory all students with acceptable entry criteria should, given an appropriate time-span and adequate feedback, be able to achieve 100%. In practice this is not usually the case, particularly where obvious time constraints exist.

Observers are sometimes surprised at the high marks that may be generated during clinical blocks, and this type of assessment may produce results which are out of line with other assessment elements commonly used in universities. Careful consideration needs to be given to how (or if) marks derived in this way should be combined with marks from more formal types of assessment in reaching an overall degree classification.

In *norm-referenced assessment*, students are compared against others in their group. A normal distribution of scores is expected and some students will fail (usually having a mark of 40% or less), while others, at the top end, will be awarded distinctions. This sort of system is commonly used in universities and enables student performance to be ranked (see Table 8.1).

Table 8.1 Comparison of norm-referenced and criterion-referenced assessment (adapted from Ewan & White 1984)

Norm-referenced	Criterion-referenced
Compares students with each other	Compares students with criterion
Students are unsure of what to learn	Students know exactly what is expected of them
Assumes learning rates are equal	Allows (ideally) for individual differences in learning rates
Might not ensure competence in essential areas	Ensures competence in essential areas
Encourages competition between students	Encourages cooperation between students
May not provide specific feedback on performance	Provides specific feedback on performance in essential areas
Maintains dependence on the educator as the arbiter of success	Develops self-direction and skills of self-assessment

Characteristics of a good assessment

Earlier in the section, the types of assessment that may be used were considered. Any method of assessment employed should fulfil certain functions:

● It should be **reliable** – two examiners assessing the same candidate or piece of work should award the same score. In clinical education, reliability can be improved by using criteria linked to explicit rating scales and by trying to ensure that all assessors are using the guidelines in the same way. Assessments using multiple choice questions (MCQs) are very reliable (as there is only one possible answer), providing the question has been well thought out. Unfortunately this form of assessment is unsuitable (lacks validity) for testing a wide range of physiotherapy skills and abilities.

- It should be **valid** – the assessment is appropriate to the task. Hence, essay writing and MCQs will not be the method of choice for assessing practical skills.
- It should be **fair** – to all students. They should all have an equal opportunity to perform well. Questions should be unambiguous and a variety of methods and markers should be used.
- It should be **practical** – in terms of time available, location, expense, etc.
- It should be **comprehensive** – testing achievement of the major objectives (the 'must know' areas) and a broad range of other important course objectives. A variety of assessment methods should be used.

In addition, the assessment should facilitate learning and contribute towards the overall course evaluation process.

ACTIVITY 8.6

Look at the example placement assessment form in Appendix 2. Consider what is being assessed and how the rating scale is constructed. Confer with more experienced assessors as to the positive and negative aspects of the use of the assessment schedule.

Warnings about assessment

- It is important, as an assessor, that you should be self-aware – the values, attitudes and beliefs that you hold may influence the assessment. It is also important to avoid bias.
- Giving a student who you know to be weak the benefit of the doubt means:
  – the learner loses out by failing to learn what it is they don't know
  – patients may lose out because standards have been compromised and may continue to be compromised in the future
  – the learner's future employing organisation(s) will aquire a weak professional
  – you have not fulfilled your professional role as an educator.
- Be aware of the 'Hawthorne' effect, i.e. changes in performance due to the student being observed.

Assessing someone else is an important task and at the end of the day you can only give an opinion based upon your experience and your expertise – guided by appropriate criteria.

Summary

This section has considered key issues relevant to assessment in the clinical setting. Here are some points to consider:

- Carry out discussions on students' requirements in private.
- Adhere as closely as possible to criteria and rating scales when these are available.
- Use the full range of the marking scale and do not refuse to give certain marks 'on principle' if they are deserved.
- Carry out feedback in private.
- Allow sufficient time for assessment and/or feedback.
- Try to discover the students' views about their own performance or progress from your discussions with them.

- When giving feedback, emphasise the positive aspects but be realistic in your criticism. It's very easy to get a reputation for consistently overrating performance and your comments will soon become devalued.
- Ensure that, at the end of your feedback, the learner is aware of their strengths and weaknesses.
- End your feedback on a positive point.

Assessment of other areas of ability have been mentioned but in-depth consideration is outside the scope of this learning package. Should you find yourself required to participate in other forms of assessment you may find some of the texts recommended in the reading package useful.

 SUMMARY ACTIVITY

List any potentially discriminatory feelings or attitudes (positive and negative) which you are able to identify in yourself in your dealings with others. These may involve appearance, lifestyle, attitudes, beliefs or personality.

Review your list and ask yourself whether your feelings could lead to bias in the way in which you assess learners.

If you have previously been in a position to assess others formally, can you identify any instance in which your marking may have been influenced by the learner's personal qualities? If so, how did you react?

REFERENCES

Block J H 1971 Introduction to mastery learning: theory and practice. In: Block J H (ed) Mastery learning: theory and practice. Holt, Rinehart and Winston, New York, ch 1

Bloom B 1956 Taxonomy of educational objectives: the classification of educational goals; Handbook one: cognitive domain. McKay, New York

Boud D 1995 Enhancing learning through self-assessment. Kogan Page, London

Caney D 1983 Competence – can it be assessed? Physiotherapy 69(9): 302–304

Cross V E M 1983 Student evaluation and assessment in clinical locations. Physiotherapy 69(9): 304–308

Ewan C, White R 1984 Teaching nursing. A self-instructional handbook. Chapman and Hall, London

Forster A L, Galley P 1978 Assessment of professional competence – the clinical teacher's responsibility. The Australian Journal of Physiotherapy 24: 53–59

Girot E A 1993 Assessment of competence in clinical practice – a review of the literature. Nurse Education Today 13: 83–90

Higher and Further Education Working Party 1979 The next decade. Council for Professions Supplementary to Medicine, London

Krathwohl D, Bloom B, Masia B 1964 A taxonomy of educational objectives: the classification of educational goals; handbook two: affective domain. McKay, New York

Quinn F M 1995 The principles and practice of nurse education. Chapman and Hall, London

Rowntree D 1987 Assessing students: How shall we know them? Kogan Page, London.

Simpson E 1972 The classification of educational objectives, in the psychomotor domain, vol. 3. Gryphin House, Washington, DC

Stoker D 1994 Assessment in learning. Methods of assessment. Nursing Times 90(13): i–viii

The Chartered Society of Physiotherapy 1991 Curriculum of study. Chartered Society of Physiotherapy, London

9

Evaluating for learning

Introduction

Throughout this package we have promoted:

- the importance of the partnership between student and educator in the process of clinical learning
- the complexity of both the clinical learning environment and the factors that influence and shape the learning that occurs there.

We now propose that both parties should continue to work together to evaluate the learning experience, and that the evaluation must acknowledge and address the complexity of the process, if it is to fulfil its purpose.

Aim

Primarily, the aim of this section is to provide the stimulus to encourage you to undertake or contribute to evaluation, and to emphasise that the activity is critical to enhancement of the learning experience and assurance of its quality.

Objectives

At the end of the section you should be able to:

1. Recognise when development and/or change in the learning experience is required.
2. Discuss the aims of undertaking an evaluation exercise.
3. Justify the time spent on this activity.
4. Work with college-based educators in planning, timing and conducting evaluation and using the information to enhance the learning experience.

How an evaluation activity might be 'triggered'

Evaluation can be 'triggered' by many different circumstances and requirements. It can also take many different forms. For example, a student discussing their placement experience with their clinical educator may state how much the opportunity to take responsibility for reporting the progress of a particular client, at a multidisciplinary team meeting, has enhanced their self-confidence and appreciation of the team approach. The educator concerned will certainly feed this back to colleagues in the clinical area and probably also to the visiting college link tutor. This should stimulate discussion as to how this aspect of the learning experience can be developed. The opinions of other students might then be sought concerning positive experiences they have had in relation to their role development to team member. This information may be obtained from face-to-face interviews, from a small questionnaire or as part of the end-of-placement evaluation.

This 'small-scale' evaluation and development can be contrasted with the activity undertaken as part of a major course review. Such reviews are needed by course management teams and are required by both the educational institution and 'purchasers' of the education programme. In this sort of evaluation, individual course modules, year programmes and overall course outcomes are reviewed. The opinions of everyone concerned with both the college-based and clinical education programmes are sought and the full range of tools to gather, analyse and interpret information is utilised.

Goals of evaluation activities

Evaluation should increase our understanding of the learning experience from the perspective of everyone concerned and enable us to implement change that will enhance the quality of teaching and learning. As professional educators, this objective is of paramount importance. However, evaluation must also be acknowledged as the means by which the quality of the educational programme is monitored. Educators are certainly not the only group who are concerned with the quality of educational provision. All parties involved in the process, including students and employers, will seek such information.

ACTIVITY 9.1

Compile a list of people, agencies or bodies that will seek to be assured of the quality of a healthcare professional education programme.

Do you think any of these will have a particular interest in the quality of the clinical education programme?

Refer back to your list as you work through this section and as the various interested parties are introduced.

Contracts and quality assurance

As previously discussed, the provision of professional education is secured by education purchasers who arrange contracts with colleges that are usually within or affiliated to the university sector. Ovretveit (1994) described three key elements of a contract. These are shown in Figure 9.1 in his diagrammatic 'contract triangle',

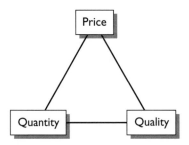

Figure 9.1 The key elements of a contract: the 'contract triangle' according to Ovretveit (1994)

in which the importance of quality is emphasised, as well as its relationship with other key elements.

Many readers will be familiar with the process of preparing, negotiating and managing service contracts. However, the application of these principles to the purchase and provision of professional education may not have been appreciated.

Many of Ovretveit's (1994) points, which were made in the context of service provision, are equally important for the 'education provider', who should both consider and address them. Consider the following examples.

A good quality system ensures that the essential elements are stated and that performance is documented. The purchaser then monitors the result – and purchasers are becoming increasingly knowledgeable about which are the better quality systems.

The incentive to specify quality is not just to be able to complete a contract specification and monitor what is done against it. Rather specifying and measuring quality is part of the process of improving quality . . . .

It will be helpful to keep in mind these ideas of evaluation as an educational, political and managerial activity as you work through the following text and activities.

Organisation of this section

In presenting this section, we are using a framework proposed by Rowntree (1986), which helps the reader to understand both the purposes and processes of evaluation.

Discussion and suggested activities will be presented under the following headings:

- What is evaluation? Why do it?
- Who is evaluation for?
- When should evaluation take place?
- How should evaluation be conducted?

What is evaluation?

Evaluation is the activity by which we find out how successful we have been in realising our educational aims, enabling students to fulfil their learning objectives, and planning, providing and facilitating the learning experience. Evaluation is concerned with what the 'course' achieves.

The processes of evaluation and assessment should be differentiated. However, these terms are quite frequently used interchangeably, especially in American literature, thus creating a potential source of confusion as to the purpose and conduct of the two activities.

Rowntree (1985) explained the difference between the two:

The difference simply is this: you assess your students but you evaluate your course. Your assessment of students will be part of the evaluation, but only part. So assessment tells you what and how well your students have learned. (p. 178)

. . . in talking of evaluating courses, [the term implies] any means by which we observe and appraise the context, the effects, and the effectiveness of the teaching and learning we have set in motion. (p. 243)

Evaluation is a rigorous procedure and, like the process of evaluating therapeutic intervention, it should stand up to the tests of scientific method.

Coles & Grant (1985) explained that evaluation is much more than just 'monitoring':

Many people quite legitimately have access to educational situations, observing what happens and passing comment on what they see, and sometimes this can lead to changes being made. But this is mere monitoring and is a somewhat amateur pursuit. An educational evaluation, however, implies judgement of merit or worth, some expression of value. The evaluator not only collects information, but also interprets, explains and makes judgements about it. Evaluators not only detect problems, for example in the way the curriculum plan works, but also attempt to explain why problems have arisen and suggest remedial action.

. . . monitoring stops at detecting the problem . . . (p. 3)

By undertaking rigorous evaluation, educators can guard against responding to anecdotal evidence. At best, this is a waste of time and energy and at worst it may actually compromise the development of the learning experience by leading us up 'blind alleys' or diverting our attention from important issues.

Although an evaluation is likely to be pre-planned and specific methods of evaluation selected, the focus of the activity can shift. In other words, the whole process may be influenced by what is discovered 'along the way'. With any human activity, and teaching and learning are very complex examples, the unexpected will frequently emerge. A good evaluation will allow for this unpredictability and permit it to have an appropriate influence on the process of development.

Consider a situation in which college-based educators are carrying out a 'routine' evaluation of students' preparedness for a specific type of clinical placement. This evaluation could take the following form:

- group feedback discussions with clinical educators
- group feedback discussions with students
- analysis of clinical progress reports, with presentation of quantitative data on student performance in clinical assessments.

Let us assume that in previous years both student and clinical educator appraisal of the placement experience has been favourable, and that student achievement has been commendable. No-one would have any reason to expect 'problems'. However, this particular evaluation reveals that all the parties involved have concerns. Students report that they felt 'out of their depth', clinical educators state that they were surprised by how much extra support students needed, and analysis of clinical assessment data reveals a drop in the standard of achievement.

There are many possible explanations for these unexpected findings. It could simply be that this particular group of students have found the placement challenging. Perhaps changes in the college-based educational experience have had a detrimental effect. Perhaps the clinical educators concerned have been working under unacceptable pressure. It is critical to discover the actual reason for such reports. Evaluators are likely to turn their attention to the individual experiences of all those concerned – students, lecturers responsible for specific course modules, clinical educators and managers – as they propose and test hypotheses.

Up until now, discussion in this section has been somewhat philosophical, in an attempt to emphasise the importance of evaluation. However, some readers will find 'models' to be a helpful way of conveying the impact that evaluation can have on the development of the learning experience.

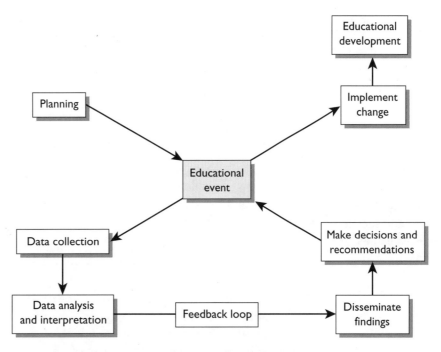

Figure 9.2 Coles & Grant's (1985) 'curriculum evaluation model'

Coles & Grant's (1985) 'curriculum evaluation model' is shown in Figure 9.2. It serves to highlight the fundamental purpose of evaluation and to emphasise its importance to the process of rational and informed decision-making.

ACTIVITY 9.2

Study Coles & Grant's 'curriculum evaluation model'. Consider it in the context of a clinical placement with which you are familiar.

Can you think of examples of activities which illustrate this 'feedback loop' in action? Was the outcome of the activity a positive one? If so, who do you feel actually derived benefit?

Evaluation – who is it for?

Students and educators

Evaluation should help to meet the needs of both students and educators. For the students, the result of evaluation should be an improvement in the quality of their learning experience and a favourable impact on their personal, professional and academic development.

The same is also true for educators. Evaluation will frequently provide them with feedback concerning the effectiveness of their teaching, and enable them to adopt a planned approach to enhancing specific teaching skills as part of their continuing professional development plan.

However, the fundamental goal of evaluation from the educator's perspective, be they college-based or clinically based, is to sustain, develop and make improvements to the 'course' on the basis of valid and reliable evidence.

Conducting an evaluation of an individual placement experience is likely to be a local initiative, but it will also be embraced in the general evaluation design and framework for the overall course programme.

ACTIVITY 9.3

What do you think it would be helpful to know about the students' perception of the quality of their learning experience?

What considerations might lead you to evaluate your own clinical teaching?

Keep these points recorded as they will prove helpful later in the chapter, in considering when and how to evaluate.

Purchasers, professional bodies, employers, universities and society as 'interested parties' in education

Evaluation is not solely for the participants in the learning process. It must also be acknowledged as a political activity, and as such it is sometimes perceived as threatening.

In the opening chapter of this package, we discussed how physiotherapy education has moved into the higher education sector and become a profession with all-graduate entry. However, the National Health Service remains the chief 'purchaser' of course places. As a result, physiotherapy course teams are accountable to various bodies, both inside and outside the university. This arrangement is shown in Figure 9.3, which also emphasises that, ultimately, we are all accountable to 'society' in the form of our clients and their carers, and any other group of people that the profession serves.

All the groups shown in Figure 9.3 will seek to be reassured that the course is both fulfilling its objectives and preparing students to meet the needs and challenges of modern healthcare. It is certainly true, however, that the various bodies may approach the process of evaluation from different perspectives and with differing priorities.

For example, the university will be very concerned with the upholding of academic standards. As well as 'routine' evaluation, internal and external audit procedures will be conducted from time to time.

The professional bodies will investigate the development of students into members of a junior healthcare team. They will also be concerned with student welfare and educational support systems. Resourcing of the course, staff–student ratios and personal tutor systems are examples of variables that will be monitored. In order to satisfy themselves, the professional bodies will carry out an initial validation prior to the start of a new course programme, followed by major review procedures at 5-yearly intervals. For both types of events, representatives from professional validation and recognition bodies will receive full-scale course documentation. In the case of review and revalidation meetings, a full course evaluation document is also required. Institutions must also arrange for the validation panel to have access to any educational facility or person involved with teaching or course management whom they wish to see. These events will always include discussions with representatives of the clinical educator group. In between revalidation events, the external examiner system ensures continuous monitoring of educational standards.

The 'purchasers' will be very concerned with how well prepared students are for current practice. They will seek to be reassured that health service managers believe that recruits from the course 'live up' to expectations. Regular educational contract reviews are conducted and clinical audit provides important information about staff efficiency and effectiveness.

All parties, but especially the professional bodies, the purchasers and students (as consumers of the educational programme), will be concerned with the quality of clinical learning experiences. Clinical education is perceived as an

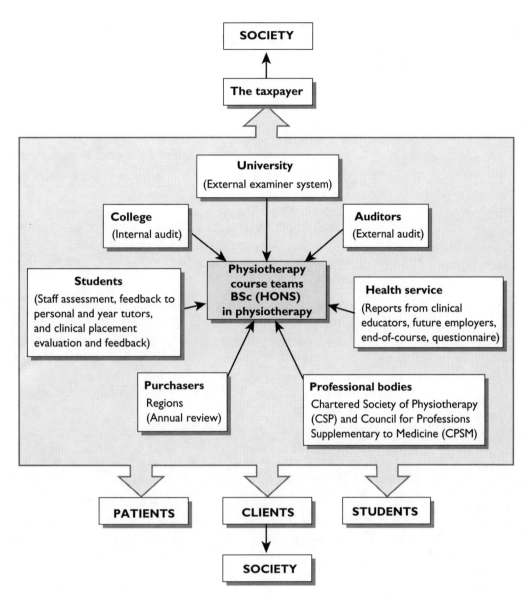

Figure 9.3 Bodies to whom physiotherapy course teams are accountable

integral and vital part of the curriculum, and as such is subject to evaluation by the course teams themselves, by external examiners who represent the professional and statutory bodies, and by representatives of the 'purchasers'. As previously mentioned, it is highly likely that you will be asked to participate in all of these evaluation exercises in your role as a clinical educator.

These examples of evaluation exercises are deliberately cited to help you to understand why educators are sometimes threatened by the process. However open we are about submitting our work for 'peer review', the implications of unfavourable feedback are never far from our minds! There is no denying the power held by 'purchasers', who in extreme cases may withdraw contracts, and by professional bodies, who may refuse to grant validation. These fortunately rare, but possible, scenarios make it even more important for those concerned with evaluation to have the skills to collect and interpret valid and reliable information. Collaborative working relationships with college-based educators, and learning environments which encourage and respect students' contributions and opinions, will do much to create an ethos of constructive feedback, evaluation and development.

ACTIVITY 9.4

Make a list of evaluation exercises specifically concerned with the quality of a clinical learning experience that either you or your colleagues have been involved in.

Who was involved in these procedures? What was the purpose of the exercise? How was feedback conveyed?

Did any tensions arise as to how the evaluation data should be used and acted upon?

The possibility of such tensions arising can be minimised, by clinical and college-based educators working collaboratively to plan, provide and evaluate the placement experience. In relation to our own (the authors) courses, we attempt to achieve this by organising:

- clinical information days, when both college- and clinically based educators present and discuss course and service developments, issues and concerns, and consider the possible impact of these on the students' clinical learning experience
- pre-clinical education planning and development meetings, where student objectives, teaching methods and assessment tools are discussed, reviewed and developed
- post-clinical education meetings, where feedback is shared and preliminary evaluation begins
- course review boards and planning meetings, which facilitate the integration of current service needs into course planning and development, and ensure that education is responding to current practice

In this spirit of collaboration, the clinical education team will make many decisions relating to the way the evaluation is conducted, the first of which will be its timing.

When to evaluate and the link with the purposes of evaluation

As previously discussed, good educators will constantly be alert to the factors influencing and shaping both the quality of the learning experience and the development of the individual learner. This ongoing activity may or may not be 'conscious' or 'deliberate', but is perceived as an integral part of the educator's role. However, as this activity frequently yields information that enables the educator to make improvements as the placement progresses, its importance and value must not be underestimated. Such evaluation is often referred to as 'formative', and as its name suggests, it is concerned with how the learning experience is developing from the perspectives of all concerned. The only cautionary note, which was mentioned previously, is that the educator should resist 'knee-jerk' responses and should constantly appraise the complexity of the learning process and the many factors that have an influence on it.

McMillan (1987) conducted a formative evaluation of a college-based nursing programme, the purposes of which were:

- to monitor the implementation of the curriculum plan
- to describe the learning environment of the students and lecturers
- to make judgements based on their feedback, so that appropriate decisions could be made about the future direction of the course.

The study revealed how a change of curriculum emphasis had caused 'upheaval' in the teaching/learning process. However, reports from the clinical educators of students who had followed the new programme were very favourable. Thus the course team maintained the courage of their convictions and 'rode through' initial difficulties.

ACTIVITY 9.5

Read the McMillan (1987) article (see Reader, p. 143) and consider the balance between informed educational decision-making and a responsiveness to students' needs. There is no easy answer to this!

Have you been encouraged to appraise a student's clinical learning experience while it was ongoing? If so, did that encouragement come from your manager or the college link tutor?

Another purpose of formative evaluation is that it may alert educators to the need for a 'full-scale' evaluation. This strategy, which is employed at the end of the placement, makes a real attempt to judge how successful the placement has been and addresses the learning experience in its entirety. It is therefore referred to as 'summative' evaluation.

ACTIVITY 9.6

What sort of events might prompt you to undertake a planned and summative evaluation of a clinical placement experience?

Can you think of an example of such an event which either you or a colleague has been involved in? Try to recall the incident(s) that prompted this action.

Such 'happenings' are sometimes referred to as critical incidents, as their analysis serves to trigger both development and change, hopefully for the better.

ACTIVITY 9.7

What experience/involvement have you had with a summative evaluation conducted at the end of a placement experience, and how was this conducted?

How should evaluation be conducted?

There exists to this day discussion, and indeed dissent, in the field of education as to how a learning experience should be evaluated and the value of the various data and feedback information.

Before we explore the various sides of this debate, it may be helpful to develop the argument concerning the differences between 'assessment' and 'evaluation'. As clinical educators are involved in both student assessment and placement evaluation, it is important to understand how both activities can provide information which will help to enhance the quality of the learning experience.

When learners are assessed, one of the aims is to discover whether they have gained knowledge, formed concepts, and acquired intellectual, practical and interpersonal skills. The 'results' should indicate whether the objectives have been achieved, but may also prompt the educator to consider whether those objectives were realistic and appropriate. Thus learner assessment can be viewed as one method, or dimension, of evaluation.

Evaluation will employ many other strategies that help in understanding the process and outcome of the learning experience. It is concerned with more than just the measurement of student achievement.

Let us look at what educationalists have to say about the multidimensional nature, importance and impact of the process of evaluation. The following quotes also serve to introduce the concept of a methodological approach to evaluation:

Evaluation is the means whereby we systematically collect and analyse information about the results of students' encounters with a learning experience. We wish to understand what it is like to teach and learn within the system we have created; to recognise which objectives have been achieved and which not; and to ascertain what unforeseen results (beneficial or disastrous) have also materialised. (Rowntree 1986, p. 192)

Evaluation is the activity by which we find out what we have been doing and how successful we have been. Without it there is little hope of improvement.

If an educator is to be in a position to understand and appraise the quality of the learning experience, and the complexities involved in the way educators and learners relate to each other in the clinical learning environment, then evaluation strategies will need to explore many aspects which may be complex in nature. It will be of little value, for example, at the end of an outpatient placement, to look at a learner's ability to examine peripheral joints, if this is the only aspect of the learning experience that is explored. Even in the context of this one aspect of therapeutic skill, there are many factors that may have impacted on an individual learner's skill development:

- Was it possible to plan a 'case load' that included people with a variety of peripheral joint problems?
- Did the learner have the opportunity to carry out both initial assessments and review?
- Did the learner have an opportunity to watch a number of therapists using various examination procedures?
- How comfortable was the learner with their clinical educator and his or her teaching strategies?
- Did the learner experience any difficulty with listening and questioning skills which may have impacted on their ability to access information?

The list is endless.

If we merely employ 'evaluation as testing' procedures, i.e. if we attempt to determine how knowledgeable and skilled the learners are at the end of the placement experience, then there is a strong possibility that we will miss the point that may truly help us to plan improvements.

An evaluator who selects tools such as preset questionnaires, attitude scales and interview schedules is operating with preconceived ideas about what is important (Cohen & Manion 1980). A college-based educator who sets up an evaluation using a pre- and post-placement experimental design will be required to fix many aspects of the conditions under which the learners (subjects) are observed. This approach has a limited ability to detect interactions. The concealed interaction may therefore 'wipe out' the main effect of the variable that chiefly concerns the investigator (Cronbach 1975).

This is not to say that these evaluation strategies are not useful in certain circumstances. However, their limitations must be fully understood and taken into account when they are employed.

It would be very wrong for the evaluator to forego the responsibility of interpreting and making judgements on the basis of available evidence. This would surely negate the value of the whole process. However, conclusions should always be preliminary, even tentative, and subject to scrutiny in subsequent placement experiences.

If the whole process of evaluation is so critical to development yet at the same time so fraught with methodological issues, how should we approach the challenge of collecting and interpreting valid and reliable information about the quality of a learning experience?

Parlett & Hamilton (1972) proposed a strategy whereby evaluation serves to 'throw light' on issues and concerns. The aims of this so-called 'illuminative evaluation' seem very appropriate in the context of clinical learning experiences. These aims are to study:

- how the programme operates
- how it is influenced by the various local situations in which it is applied
- what are its advantages and disadvantages, according to those directly concerned
- how students' learning tasks and experiences are influenced and shaped
- what it is like to be either a learner or an educator participating in the learning experience.

In summary, such approaches seek to address and illuminate a complex array of questions.

Illuminative evaluation is described by its designers and supporters as 'not a standard methodological package but a general research strategy'. However, there are two methodological features that must be addressed by those attempting this sort of approach. First, no method is used in isolation – different techniques are combined to throw light on a common problem. One of the advantages of this procedure, known as triangulation, is that tentative findings can be cross-checked. Secondly, the evaluation must follow three distinct but overlapping phases. Evaluators will observe, inquire further, and then seek to explain. Prior specification of a detailed evaluation plan is inappropriate, as the approach deliberately allows for the unanticipated to emerge.

Finally, we use the words of the promoters of this type of evaluation to convey the philosophy underpinning this approach:

[In illuminative evaluation] attempted measurement of educational products is abandoned for intensive study of the program as a whole: its rationale and evolution, its operations, achievement and difficulties . . . .

Observations, interviews with participants (students, instructors, administrators and others), questionnaires, and analysis of documents and background information are all combined to help 'illuminate' problems, issues and significant program features.

In Box 9.1, adapted from Harris & Bell (1986), some of the methods and means of collecting information and evidence for the purposes of evaluation are listed, under the following headings:

- listening and talking techniques
- observation
- paper and pencil techniques.

Box 9.1 Means of collecting information

---

1 LISTENING AND TALKING TECHNIQUES

- **Informal discussions**

Arising spontaneously, these may prove a good 'starting point' for collecting information, i.e. they may form the basis for further investigations. Such discussions may be conducted:
  - one-to-one
  - in groups

- **Interviews**

When interviews are conducted, the investigator/evaluator has a definite need or purpose in collecting information. Skill is involved in both conducting the interview and recording findings. Research methodology texts will help you with these issues. Interviews may be:
  - **structured**: when particular questions are asked, with little opportunity for the interviewee to raise issues of their own
  - **partially structured:** where the interviewee has much more opportunity to contribute to the 'agenda' of the conversation. Such interviews are particularly helpful in meeting both the needs of the learner (to raise issues) and the educator (to maintain focus)
  - **non-structured:** carefully planned, conducted with a purpose and therefore very different from the spontaneous informal discussions previously described. Experience and skill is required for successful conduct of such interviews and the 'new' evaluator should consider a more structured approach to interviewing. In experienced hands, the non-structured interview may reveal information and provide insight in a way that other 'techniques' have failed to do

- **Group discussions**

These have the advantage of accessing information and gaining feedback from a larger number of people. A 'good' group will develop ideas and may even come towards solutions to problems through problem-solving. However, the skill of the group leader is very important. Most groups will need either some structure or facilitation. This may be achieved by:
  - **snowball technique:** group members work independently to begin with and record their responses to, and feelings about, a particular issue. Group activity is built up by progressive sharing, pooling and then summarising perspectives, first in pairs, then in small groups, until a full group discussion ensues
  - **brainstorming:** all members of the group are invited to record their initial responses to a particular issue or concern. All responses are accepted and valued. The whole group then engages in organisation and synthesis of material and the process of formulating conclusions or identifying the need for further information
  - **buzz groups:** a large group divides into small groups of no more than four people, in order to focus attention, through discussion, on a particular issue. As a result, the groups are considerably better able to contribute to a whole-group, or plenary, discussion session

2 OBSERVATION

Healthcare professionals are skilled observers and may usefully transfer this skill to the observation of learners in action in the clinical setting. Naturally, considerable interpersonal skill is required to carry out this activity with sensitivity and respect for both the student and their patient. Observation may be

- **Structured**

This is an especially useful technique when more 'open' procedures have revealed an issue that is worthy of further investigation. Focus is maintained and pertinent information collected

- **Non-structured**

As is the case for non-structured interviewing, this procedure allows for the 'unexpected' to emerge, and may provide both rich and insightful information. However, the same cautions apply – the non-structured approach is not for the 'new' evaluator

3 PENCIL AND PAPER TECHNIQUES

- **Using assessments**

As previously discussed, assessment information forms *part* of evaluation and should be regularly collected, presented and analysed

- **Use of questionnaires**

A clinical placement evaluation questionnaire is frequently designed by the educational institution. An example is given in Appendix 3. Questionnaires have the advantage of collecting, relatively quickly, information from a large number of people. However, their design is critical to the quality of the information obtained. Interested readers are strongly advised to refer to research methodology texts on this subject

- **Delphi techniques**

In this technique, information is collected from a group using various methodologies. It is then collated, analysed and summarised by the investigator. Information from the summary is then fed back to the group, which hopefully generates further comment

- **Diaries**

These are written records of events from the perspective of the learner. The introduction to the 'professional development diary' should promote the use of such valuable insights in the process of evaluation

These methods will be used in different combinations depending on the individual context and the particular study.

ACTIVITY 9.8

Review the list of methods of collecting evaluative information and evidence. How many of these techniques are you familiar with? You may wish to obtain additional information on those you have not heard of before.

Those of you who have undertaken courses on research methods are likely to be familiar with such approaches, and your experience will be highly valued in the process of planning evaluation studies. However, in the spirit and philosophy of illuminative evaluation, the opinions and experiences of everyone contributing to, and participating in, the learning experience are considered to be important, if appropriate judgements about improvement and development are to be made.

ACTIVITY 9.9

Return to the factors that you identified in Activity 9.3 as 'triggers' to evaluating the quality of either the learning experience or your teaching in your role as clinical educator. What means of collecting information might help you to understand more about the 'problem' you have identified?

How might you reconcile the need to make judgements that will inform the development of the clinical placement learning experience with the need constantly to appraise the validity of your own conclusions?

Final thoughts

You may have wondered initially why this section is entitled 'Evaluating *for* learning' instead of simply 'Evaluating learning'. Harris & Bell (1986) contend that the concept of evaluation is vital within the context of current adult learning theories.

It has been our intention also to promote evaluation as an integral part of course design and development, and therefore as being inextricably linked with the assurance of quality of learning. It is a cooperative venture for educators and students, and should be undertaken in the spirit of collaboration and respect for the student as an adult and self-directed learner.

Summary

In this section, you have been introduced to evaluation as a critical element of successful course design and development.

Various approaches to evaluation have been reviewed. You are encouraged to appraise them for their value and relevance to the process of developing clinical education programmes.

It is hoped that you will now feel able to participate in evaluation activities, carefully selecting and reviewing the various methods of collecting information with regard to their validity and reliability in informing the development of the clinical learning experience.

REFERENCES

Cohen L, Manion L 1980 Research methods in education. Croom Helm, London

Coles C R, Grant J G 1985 Curriculum evaluation in medical and health care education. ASME Medical Education Research Booklet No. 1. Medical Education 19: 405.

Cronbach L J 1975 Beyond two disciplines of scientific psychology. American Psychologist 30: 116–127

Harris D, Bell C 1986 Evaluating and assessing for learning. Kogan Page, London

McMillan M A 1987 An illuminative approach to a formative evaluation of a college-based nursing program. Nurse Education Today 7: 156–170

Ovretveit J 1994 Physiotherapy service contracts and 'business autonomy'. Physiotherapy 80(6): 372–376

Parlett M, Hamilton D 1972 Evaluation as illumination: a new approach to the study of innovatory programs. Occasional Paper, October 1972. University of Edinburgh, Centre for Research in the Educational Sciences, Edinburgh

Rowntree D 1985 Developing courses for students, 2nd edn. Harper and Row, London

Rowntree D 1986 Educational technology in curriculum development, 2nd edn. Harper and Row, London

10 The development and purpose of clinical education

Introduction

This self-directed learning pack began by placing clinical education into the context of the overall physiotherapy educational process and by considering some of the contemporary factors in the changing health and education scene that are having an impact on this process. As with all aspects of the profession, clinical education has changed over time, and it is this development which will be considered in this section.

Aim

This section aims to help you consider more carefully the development and purpose of clinical education and to raise your awareness of some additional dimensions to its importance in the overall education process. In-depth consideration of these dimensions is beyond the scope of this practical workbook, but readers who are interested in particular issues are urged to follow up the references in the articles quoted below. Additional reading such as this will enhance the material already covered in this pack and generate an even greater understanding of the complexities of clinical education.

Some of the more recent professional developments related to clinical education are also referred to in this section.

Objectives

By the end of this section you should have a raised awareness of:

1. The historical development of clinical education, including some recent professional developments which support the clinical education process.
2. The multi-faceted purpose of clinical education for learners, in both the short and long term.
3. Current policy issues impacting on health professional education.
4. Specific post-registration and continuing clinical education matters.

An outline of the historical developments of pre-registration physiotherapy education with particular reference to clinical education

An appreciation of the early history of the profession is both interesting and helpful for putting today's clinical education challenges into an appropriate context. The history is well documented by Wicksteed (1948), Barclay (1994) and Thornton

(1994). Physiotherapy education today can trace its roots directly to the endeavours of a small group of qualified nurses and midwives in the 1890s. They sought to protect their skills of 'medical rubbing', which was already well accepted in medicine for a range of conditions, from the unscrupulous practitioners responsible for the 'massage scandal' of 1894. The scandal, which involved Scotland Yard and the Home Secretary (later Prime Minister), Herbert Asquith, was reported in the British Medical Journal of the time, and is recounted by Barclay (1994). As a consequence, and to protect bona fide practitioners, the Society of Trained Masseuses was founded in 1895. The founders were really the first mature students of the profession, as most were already qualified nurses and/or midwives. Some had trained at the London Hospital and developed their massage skills on the job, while others were taught massage by doctors, either in hospitals or in schools of massage, or by private tuition.

By 1900, the Society of Trained Masseuses, which was already a governing body, became the Incorporated Society of Trained Masseuses, thereby gaining greater official and legal status. However, it was not until 1913 that it became an essential requirement for all students preparing for the massage examination to 'see, and give under supervision, treatments to actual patients in hospitals, infirmaries or equivalent cliniques during their training' (Wicksteed 1948). Interestingly, Wicksteed noted problems relating to the availability of placements and remuneration for the clinical supervisors, which are familiar today. She reported that the 'Council acknowledged that the difficulties of arranging this [supervision] would be great, especially in the provinces' and that the students usually paid an additional fee to the Society of 2/6d (12½p) per month, which was used to pay the supervisors.

However, apart from this requirement there was no standard for training because as it was recognised that 'some people learn faster than others although 6 months is always advocated . . .' (Wicksteed 1948). At that time, the training was still undertaken in a variety of ways, including by private tuition and individual coaching.

The increased demand for practitioners that arose in the First World War led to a postponement of plans by the Council and teachers to extend the length of training, although by necessity new material was introduced to the syllabus and the courses became more demanding, with examinations in medical electricity being introduced in 1915.

By 1920, the shortage of recognised teachers had become so acute that some schools were under threat of closure. This situation led four training schools to send their pupils to universities for the theoretical components of the course, to be taught by doctors. In the same year, the Society was granted its Royal Charter and merged with the Institute of Massage and Medical Gymnastics. The merged body became known as the Chartered Society of Massage and Medical Gymnastics. Under the terms of the Charter, the Society was established as the only recognised examining and professional body for physiotherapists in the United Kingdom, and was authorised to 'promote a curriculum and standard of qualification for persons engaged in the practice of massage, medical gymnastics, electrotherapeutics and kindred methods of treatment' (Royal Charter, Chartered Society of Massage and Medical Gymnastics 1920). To this end, in 1927, the first conjoint examinations in massage and Swedish remedial exercises were introduced, thus establishing a minimum national qualification.

With the evacuation of many cities and the government ban on large gatherings during the Second World War, students were dispersed throughout the country, but their training and examinations continued uninterrupted throughout the war period, despite considerable difficulties. Meeting the needs of war casualties highlighted shortcomings in the existing syllabus and set the foundation stones for the Chartered Society of Physiotherapy, as it became known in 1943, to develop a 3-year syllabus. This syllabus, which was introduced nationally in 1947, contained theoretical and clinical components and 3 weeks nursing experience. It covered massage, exercise therapy, electrotherapy and rehabilitation. The clinical component was a minimum of 750 hours, although this was later doubled to 1500 hours, to be reduced to the present 1000 hours in 1976. There were three examinations during the course and one included practical skills tests, but these were all undertaken on models or examiners. The third, final exam was a role play of the treatment of three (later two) different cases, with the part of the patient being acted out by a junior student who, if they had not already covered the condition in their training, would lack the necessary knowledge and experience to act convincingly.

Around the time of the establishment of the NHS in 1948, a number of new schools attached to teaching hospitals opened. Throughout the country, the role of the clinical educators, or supervisors as they were then known, had continued to develop as had their contribution to the various national examination systems which followed, but all pre-registration courses were run in NHS schools of physiotherapy and students received the majority of their clinical education from the group of teaching hospitals to which the school was attached. Moreover, many Principals of the schools of physiotherapy were also the service Group Superintendents.

In 1976, 56 years after the first students had lectures, the first university degree course was introduced, although it was to be another 16 years before physiotherapy became an all-graduate entry profession, in 1992; the last round of national examinations was held in 1993. During this time of transition, there was a marked development in the contribution of the clinical physiotherapist to the education of students, as their role developed from one of supervising the clinical caseload of a number of students to that of a skilled clinical educator, usually working on a one-to-one or one-to-two basis. Furthermore, their precise role in, and contribution to, the universities' examination process is now course-specific, and the skills required to undertake this complex role successfully are many and varied, as we have identified throughout this package.

The major service changes of the last decade, coupled with changing demands in the higher education sector, will no doubt be reflected in the Society's current curriculum review. The impact of this remains to be seen, as does the outcome of current debates about such human resource issues as skill mix, specialists crossing professional boundaries, generic workers and national vocational qualifications. These debates will help to shape the next chapter in the history of clinical education.

ACTIVITY 10.1

Read Cross's (1994) review paper 'From clinical supervisor to clinical educator: too much to ask?' (See Reader, p. 149.)

In various activities throughout this pack, you have been asked to reflect upon your own clinical education experiences as a student. Now consider where these experiences fit in Cross's spiral model of the development of physiotherapy practice and clinicians' roles in clinical education.

Consider also the resources you have drawn on to help with your own personal development as a clinical educator.

Recent professional developments related to pre-registration clinical education

From 1989, the pending introduction of the NHS reforms, with the various contracting processes, led members to call upon the Society to set national standards for physiotherapy practice that could be universally adopted and used by services locally to set and review standards of practice. In 1990, in response, the Society issued the first ever national standards of practice for physiotherapy. These standards were primarily concerned with areas of clinical practice, and the various clinical interest groups contributed to their production. However, in 1991, a further document, 'Standards for clinical education placements' (The Chartered Society of Physiotherapy 1991a), was introduced. This sought to identify good practices in relation to the organisation and running of clinical placements, and was drawn up to offer a framework to academic staff and service managers for negotiating placements and to act as a common reference for clinical educators and students on placements alike.

ACTIVITY 10.2

Read the 'Standards for clinical education placements' document. Is this the first time you have read it?

If you are a clinical educator, assess your own contribution towards the maintenance of the standards, and identify the mechanisms you have for auditing the continuing application of the standards.

Are these mechanisms adequate? How do you judge whether this is the case?

A further development of the document on standards was the recognition by the Society's education committee of the need to draw up a policy whereby appropriate standards of placements were ensured without threatening their continuing supply. To this end, in 1992, the committee established the 'Clinical Education Working Party', which produced 'Guidelines for good practice for the education of clinical educators' (The Chartered Society of Physiotherapy 1994), published early in 1994. These guidelines, which were produced following consultation with managers and course leaders, contained indicative rather than mandatory recommendations, and sought to facilitate placements and were designed to be used in conjunction with the standards document. In recognition of the complexities of clinical education, the working party emphasised the need for specific education for the clinical educators, and identified and promoted two types of training that were desirable. Programmes which cover the broad educational issues needed in workplace teaching and supervision were identified as type A, and could, if suitable, be PACE accredited (see later) and/or multidisciplinary, while those which deal directly with a specific course, and the relationship between the course and its placement providers, were identified as type B.

Another dimension in the clinical education equation which has been problematic for many years is the 'Clinical supervisors' allowance' which is part of the Whitley Council agreement. This allowance, which is paid to clinical educators, was traditionally funded from within the budget of the placement provider, usually from other savings, and was only very rarely funded from source. However, the introduction of the market economy in the NHS, the move of physiotherapy education into the higher education sector and the prospect of the implementation of locally agreed reward strategies are all factors which have, in the early 1990s, conspired to generate fresh interest in the allowance. The Society and other professional bodies recognise the difficulties arising from historical precedents, but their resolution and the future of the allowance are matters that are inextricably linked with the future of Whitley Council and the introduction of local pay agreements.

The development of post-registration physiotherapy education

The founders met together in London, where the massage scandal was centred, and so the Society's roots are in the capital. However, the profession grew quickly, as did the demand for the decentralisation of facilities (in particular examinations), most notably from Manchester, where an independent society was rapidly growing, with its own training programmes and examinations. This was quickly followed by a demand for lectures to be arranged outside London, and again, Manchester was to the fore, being the first other city to house a regional centre for the Society. Here, lectures were given, meetings held and library facilities made available. By 1920 when the Royal Charter was granted, there were lecture centres established in Bournemouth, Dublin, Edinburgh, Glasgow, Liverpool and Manchester. The Charter made provision for the formation of local boards: 'they were instituted by Council in order to guard the interests of all members in the area which they served, be a means of spreading knowledge of the Society, and form a liaison between the local medical practitioners and the Society' (Wicksteed 1948). However, this did not obviate the members' demand for local lecture centres, and by 1926 the Society resolved to establish branches on a local geographical basis and with a standard constitution.

By the time the NHS was established in 1948, the geographical structure of the various boards and branches almost matched that of the regional hospital boards. The Society's boards ran their own congresses, study weekends and post-registration courses. This membership structure has remained to the present day, although there is now increasing concern about whether this is still the best way to serve the members and the Society. In particular, there is circumstantial evidence that the decrease in demand for post-registration education through the branch network is related to the increase in the strength of specific interest groups and district-based services with in-service training programmes. Given the present demise of district services, it will be interesting to see if this remains the case.

The first specific interest groups were occupational ones formed to promote the interest of their members, but in 1945 the Association of Orthopaedic Physiotherapists was established for practitioners who were both physiotherapists and orthopaedic nurses. This was followed in 1948 by the Obstetrics Physio-therapists Association which was formed, among other things, to share knowledge. Other clinical interest groups formed and gradually took on the responsibility for promoting expertise, experience and continuing education in their specific areas of practice, through conferences, journals, lectures and other study programmes with theoretical and practical components. The Manipulation Association of Chartered Physiotherapists was the first to push the post-registration clinical education frontier forward when, in 1979, after 7 years of preparation, it implemented a standard requirement for membership of '100 hours of supervised training and 200 hours of supervised clinical work on the vertebral column and 60 and 150 hours, respectively, on peripheral joints' (Barclay 1994).

Since then, many other specific interest groups have developed post-registration courses with a significant clinical component, which the learners undertake either as supervised field-work in their own service or on placement to the service of their senior clinical educator. Throughout the 1970s, recognition of the need for continuing post-registration education grew, and in recognition of the endeavours of all the course organisers and their participants, the Society developed a system of validation for post-registration courses. By 1985, ten courses had been validated and twelve more were being planned.

In the late 1980s, the Society entered into a consultative programme with members to seek their views on requirements for post-registration education. This resulted in the publication of its 'Post-registration education master plan' (Titchen 1988), and as a result of further consultation with members, the Post-registration Education Working Party devised the 'Physiotherapy access to continuing education' (PACE) scheme to provide a structure for continuing education for all UK physiotherapists. The aim of the scheme was to encourage all individual practitioners to continue their professional learning throughout their career through a credit-based system of study. However, the PACE development coincided with the consolidation of pre-registration education into the higher education sector and the proliferation of the many varied and flexible opportunities in higher education for diplomates and graduates alike, including greater access to research and educational expertise, Masters and other higher degree programmes, and other multidisciplinary learning opportunities. Hence, within a short period the PACE scheme was expanded and will be the subject of a further major review by the Society in 1995–1996.

One ambitious element of the PACE system was to credit an individual's demonstrated experiential learning, thereby recognising aspects of their clinical practice. As part of this process, the learner was required to maintain a portfolio of their experience which could be wide-ranging in content. A specific tool was developed for this purpose, which became known as the 'professional development diary'. The value of maintaining a career diary was quickly and generally accepted, and this tool was in turn further developed for use both inside and outside the PACE system by pre- and post-registration learners.

A further development from this in the 1990s has been the growing recognition and acceptance of the need for continuing professional development (CPD) as 'a way of ensuring that members are keeping up to date professionally and enhancing their competence which should, in turn, benefit patient care' (O'Sullivan 1995). By the autumn of 1995, all members received a leaflet from the Society promoting the concept of CPD and identifying a number of key activities to be conducted on a regular and systematic basis throughout their working life, in line with the principles of analysis, action plan and review.

The purpose of clinical education

Section 1 referred to the CSP's 1991 Curriculum of Study for pre-registration undergraduate physiotherapy programmes and acknowledged the vital place of clinical education in the overall physiotherapy education process. While the specific requirements of different areas of postgraduate clinical education are different, the underlying principles are not.

Clinical education is an essential and indispensable course element which provides the focus for the integration of the knowledge and skills learnt at the college base.
(The Chartered Society of Physiotherapy 1991b)

The core curriculum continues to stipulate:

One thousand (1000) hours of clinical education is considered the minimum amount needed to achieve an acceptable level of competence. Successful completion of the clinical education component is required.

ACTIVITY 10.3

At the time of writing, the CSP was undertaking a review of the 1991 core curriculum. Check whether this has been superseded as yet.

If it has, compare the section on clinical education in the latest core curriculum with the 1991 version. Seek to discuss any differences with colleagues, including if possible the visiting tutor from any physiotherapy course to which your service offers placements.

The specification of 1000 hours of clinical education for pre-registration physiotherapists is rooted in the history of the profession, but it means that the clinical education component represents approximately one-third of the total course, regardless of the individual course design and structure. Comparison with pre-registration physiotherapy courses in other industrialised countries shows this to be about average.

As was described in the Brook (1994) article you read in activity 1.1, every UK undergraduate physiotherapy course is now unique in its philosophy, curriculum structure and course design, yet as we see from the core curriculum, all have to fulfil the requirement of a minimum of 1000 hours of clinical education throughout the total length of the course. As the 1991 core curriculum specifies, this is to ensure the integration of academic and practical knowledge and skills. Inseparable from that is the development of personal attitudes and beliefs and the start of professional life.

Clearly, this integration process can be undertaken satisfactorily in a number of ways, otherwise there would not be such a wide range of acceptable structures of clinical education programmes within physiotherapy courses.

ACTIVITY 10.4

Look at the pattern of clinical placements within the overall course structure of all physiotherapy courses which have places commissioned by your region. This will be found in the course documents.

Compare the different patterns and think of each in terms of the implications for, and impact on, the learners, educators and your own service.

The integration process

This integration process, which goes on throughout an undergraduate's clinical education programme, marks the beginning of their transition from pure academic to expert practitioner and involves much more than the reformulation of applied theoretical knowledge and the consolidation of clinical skills in a variety of learning environments, with all the complexities examined in Section 6. Some of the additional dimensions of this process are discussed in the following sections.

In the actual text of the core curriculum, the purpose of clinical education seems straightforward, and we have used the previous sections of this pack to consider how to achieve successfully the 'integration' which the core curriculum so neatly describes. But why is it necessary? What does this integration process involve?

Dictionaries vary in their definition of integration, but here are some from the *Penguin English Dictionary* which are useful in this context:

- *harmonious combination of elements into a complex whole*
- *removal of social barriers between previously segregated groups*
- *development and unification of awareness.*

Keeping abreast of service demands

Morris (1993), in examining three current approaches to medical and physiotherapy undergraduate education, stated the following frank opinion:

Graduates also need to function as competent and effective professionals in the real world and not simply possess academic knowledge. Physiotherapy has an academic base but it requires practitioners who are able to apply their knowledge.

Furthermore, she held the view that:

Concern with course design and undergraduate education is of interest to clinicians as well as to educators because clinical staff are often involved with students on clinical placements and the students' school education will affect their clinical performance.

This involvement has reciprocal advantages because, as has been the case throughout the development of the profession, it is clinicians who are best placed to identify changing service needs and who will develop new clinical practices in response to these changes. Learners on placements in a range of service settings will informally witness this dimension of the process without necessarily recognising it as such. Therefore, it is the clinicians' responsibility to keep the educators informed about new clinical trends, thereby helping to ensure that education remains commensurate with changing service and thus with employers' needs.

This is normally done formally through representative clinicians serving on relevant course committees, and more informally through liaison between clinicians and the academic visiting tutor. In this text, we have deliberately refrained from making significant reference to the visiting tutor because it is clear that their role and the nature of their visits is course-specific. For example, in some institutions the visiting tutor is actively involved in the assessment process and in teaching, whereas in others the visiting tutor's role is purely one of liaison.

Being at the frontiers of clinical practice

This tendency has been well illustrated throughout the history of the profession, from the time when the founders of the physiotherapy profession undertook to take positive action about the massage scandal of 1894 and launched the Society of Trained Masseuses. In the early days of the Industrial Revolution, the names of major hospitals alone were sufficient to identify the main aspects of their workload and the clinical experience to be gained therein. The London, Midland and Scottish Railway Hospital at Crewe and The Royal Victoria and Albert Dock Hospital on the Thames are just two examples of names that reflected the nature of the industrial injury caseloads from the new industries of railways and docks.

A contemporary example of clinical practice guiding educational practice in the development of new material is in the advancement of physiotherapy clinical practices in the management of patients with HIV and AIDS. This is well illustrated by Lang (1993) in her case study 'Community physiotherapy for people with HIV/AIDS'. Lang recognises that 'awareness of the possible role of physiotherapy does not appear to be high among physiotherapists themselves' and she calls for greater research into the role of the community practitioner, and identifies, given the changing nature of the condition, the need for the exchange of information about knowledge and practice between the different specialities.

Having the opportunity to formulate one's own health and other social beliefs

Entry into any clinical learning environment immediately exposes the learner to a host of new encounters, and by sampling the range of health beliefs of others, and the various cultural differences in the responses to therapeutic intervention that are found within the population, the learner is able to develop their own health beliefs further. This may also involve the chance to reassess earlier personal experiential learning as a recipient of healthcare. Synthesising such experiences can enrich a developing clinician in the long term but may well be the cause of additional concerns in the short term.

In particular, the recent growth of the lobby for the rights of people with disabilities has provided much thought-provoking literature for therapy health professionals to consider. This gives a clear indication that it is not only learners, but also many experienced practitioners, who need to develop their health beliefs further. To illustrate how successful this movement has been in raising awareness and getting their issues onto the education agenda, Johnson (1993, Research project, BSc Hons Physiotherapy), when considering the implications for clinical practice, claimed:

> *If departmental discussions and investigations of client perceptions can lead to better therapeutic relationships, then physiotherapists as well as patients can only benefit.*

She concluded:

> *Comprehensive disability awareness training should be part of every physiotherapy education curriculum. [. . .] this should be conducted by disabled people to challenge attitudes and present more positive views.*

Facing moral and ethical issues and clinical decision-making

Gaining experience on clinical placements enables learners to acquire the necessary attributes to develop their clinical judgement in order to practice efficiently and effectively. Emphasis on this has grown over the last 20 years or so, along with the development of professional autonomy. Simultaneously, with advancing technology, raised patient and carer expectations and, latterly, some business considerations, the range of moral and ethical issues facing health practitioners has also grown. Junior learners may be sufficiently challenged by a simple either/or clinical decision, but as their experience deepens they will find themselves increasingly confronting moral and ethical issues which impact on their clinical decision-making. This whole field is rich in complexities but it is clear that it should be addressed by every practitioner:

> *. . . professional treatment decisions must be based on ethical analysis; ethical decision making must take place as a component of clinical decision making. Development of the ability to make ethical decisions is an essential component of professional growth; without ethical decision making, the treatment decisions made by physical therapists have the potential to jeopardise the advancement of the profession.'* (Clawson 1994)

Current policy issues impacting on health professional education

Section 1 outlined the national policy and process of commissioning pre-registration physiotherapy education that was in place at the time of writing (1994). It was pointed out that this was likely to alter with the implementation of the changes to regional health authorities.

ACTIVITY 10.5

Find out whether any changes to the policy and the commissioning process have occurred as yet, and if so what they are, and whether there have been any other relevant central policy changes.

Education news items and reports to Council in the Physiotherapy Journal will be useful sources of information if you have difficulty accessing the latest relevant NHSE Letters. Moreover, there may be physiotherapy managers in your service who are involved in informing service providers about their commissioning requirements.

Summary

Cross (1994) provides the final, appropriately concluding, activity for this section. A time for completion of the activity is not specified, because if you have worked through this pack thus far, you are likely to have considered the issue already, either consciously or subconsciously.

 SUMMARY ACTIVITY

Read the Cross (1994) article again (Reader, p. 149) and consider the question she poses in her final paragraph: is it too much to ask clinicians to accept and fulfil the role of clinical educator at this time?

As a group of physiotherapists we (the authors) also feel it is a vital question, and one which has underpinned our motivation to write this pack. We hope this pack will be of some help in equipping you to answer the question, thereby enabling you to contribute more fully to determining the future direction of the profession.

Having completed the pack thus far, you will be better placed to make that contribution through your role as a clinical educator and you may have speculated on ideas for future developments.

Completion of the next section will enable you to assess your progress and to reflect upon your own development in this role since starting the pack.

REFERENCES

Barclay J 1994 In good hands, 1st edn. Butterworth Heinemann, Oxford

Clawson A L 1994 The relationship between clinical decision making and ethical decision making. Physiotherapy 80(1): 10–14

Cross V 1994 From clinical supervisor to clinical educator: too much to ask? Physiotherapy 80(9): 609–611

Johnson R 1993 Attitudes don't just hang in the air. Physiotherapy 79(9): 619-627

Lang C 1993 Community physiotherapy for people with HIV/AIDS. Physiotherapy 79(3): 163–167

Morris J 1993 An overview of and comparison among three current approaches to medical and physiotherapy undergraduate education. Physiotherapy 79(2): 91–94

O'Sullivan J 1995 Continuing professional development. Chartered Society of Physiotherapy, London

The Chartered Society of Massage and Medical Gymnastics (later The Chartered Society of Physiotherapy) 1920 Royal Charter. Chartered Society of Massage and Medical Gymnastics, London

The Chartered Society of Physiotherapy 1991a Standards for clinical education placements. Chartered Society of Physiotherapy, London

The Chartered Society of Physiotherapy 1991b Curriculum of study. Chartered Society of Physiotherapy, London

The Chartered Society of Physiotherapy 1994 Guidelines for good practice for the education of clinical educators. Chartered Society of Physiotherapy, London

Thornton E 1994 100 years of physiotherapy education. Physiotherapy 80(A): 11A–19A

Titchen A C 1988 The development of the post-registration education master plan. Physiotherapy 74(1): 10–12

Wicksteed J 1948 The growth of a profession, 1st edn. Arnold & Co., London

11 The learning experience model in action: consolidatory self-assessment exercises

Introduction

Having completed the first 10 sections of this package, you now have all the tools necessary to plan, design, implement, assess and evaluate a learning experience for either a group of learners or an individual learner. Now gather together all of the notes and responses you have made in completing the activities in Sections 1–10. These will be useful to you as you work through this section.

This section is designed to help you to integrate all you have learned throughout the package and to plan a complete learning experience for learners for whom you have responsibility in your professional life.

You may have planned learning experiences in the past, but in completing the following exercises, we hope that you will broaden your planning skills, develop new ideas to aid the learning process and feel increased confidence in both the assessment and evaluation of a learning experience. Thus, we hope that you will feel able to participate more fully in all stages of a successful learning experience.

During this section, you will familiarise yourself with the curriculum development model, put stages of the model into action hypothetically, and then you will be encouraged to use the complete model in practice. There is no need to complete all the activities in one go; work at your own pace, according to when there is time available and when the opportunity arises in the workplace to carry out the activities in relation to events that are taking place.

Aim

By using the curriculum model provided, this section aims to enable you to design, implement, assess and evaluate a complete learning experience and, in doing so, include the following key stages:

1. Assess learner entry behaviour.
2. Assess and agree learning objectives.
3. Plan and design a learning experience.
4. Implement the learning experience.
5. Assess learning outcomes.
6. Evaluate the learning experience.
7. Reflect on the whole learning process and implement change at appropriate stages of the cycle, if required.

The curriculum model

The model in Figure 11.1 (after Rowntree 1982) shows a typical curriculum development cycle. The term 'curriculum' relates to the design of a total learning

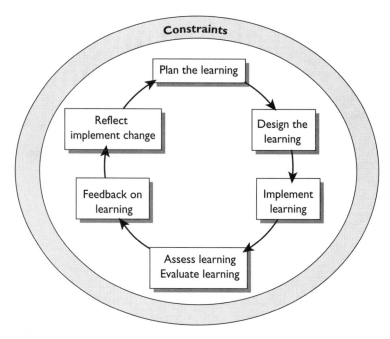

Figure 11.1 Curriculum development model (after Rowntree 1982)

experience. This model can be adapted for many needs. It has been adapted here to complement the design process for clinical education placements or other learning experience planning which you may be involved in.

The model consists of a central core which is surrounded by a ring of constraints. Within the constraints of any curriculum design, a number of events take place in a cyclic and interactive fashion. They are represented in this model by the six stages within the inner circle. These stages are:

- planning the learning
- designing the learning
- implementing the learning
- evaluating the learning
- obtaining feedback on the learning
- reflecting on the learning process.

It will be useful now to consider more thoroughly each stage of the cycle, but before doing so we suggest that you revisit your perceptions of your role as a clinical educator and, in particular, reflect on the 'OK behaviours' you would wish to bring to this learning experience, and on how you intend to deal with or modify any 'not-OK behaviours' you have identified in yourself. Refer back to Section 2 and to the Davis & McKain (1975) article to refresh your memory of the behaviours associated with the clinical educator's role.

The stages of the model will be described in terms of a clinical education placement for a student physiotherapist, but the principles can be adapted for use in any learning situation.

Constraints

Any learning experience occurs within the context of constraints, which may be of an environmental, attitudinal, political, managerial or personal nature.

ACTIVITY 11.1

Taking your own working environment as an example, list all the constraints that exist which may affect the implementation of a clinical education placement.

You may have listed some of the following factors: your non-educational responsibilities in the workplace, time that is available for clinical teaching, the level of entry behaviour of the learner, the availability of suitable patients for a learner's caseload, the environment in which learning is to take place, learner/staff motivation, your (as an educator) and your colleagues' commitment to an education programme and irregularities in the transportation services bringing patients to the clinical education setting. The list is endless.

ACTIVITY 11.2

Now analyse the effects each of the constraints you have listed may have on the learning experience.

Specifically, constraints can be divided up into:

1. those which affect the individual student
2. those which affect the educator
3. those which affect the running of the department in which the clinical education placement is based
4. organisational constraints such as internal politics, financial arrangements and staffing levels.

All of these may be beyond the control of the learner and/or the educator, but they will have profound effects on the quality of any clinical placement.

ACTIVITY 11.3

Take your original list of constraints and place them into one of the four categories listed above. Doing so may highlight factors which you have missed. Make sure you consider each category carefully and analyse the effect of any further constraints you add to the list.

Discuss your list of constraints with colleagues who may think of some more additions.

Now consider if there are any ways in which the constraints on the list may be modified in order to reduce their impact on the learning experience. This modification may not always be possible, but the exercise can be fruitful in terms of rationalising the size of the proposed obstacles.

Planning the learning experience

During this stage in the cycle, the educator needs to be able to describe the learner's entry behaviour, plan local placement objectives in relation to entry behaviour, plan the implementation of the learning process, plan assessment procedures relative to the objectives that have been set, and consider how the placement will be evaluated in the long and short terms. At this stage you will not as yet have met the learner, so you need to be prepared to modify your plans at the beginning of the placement when an individual's learning needs become clearer. See Section 3 for a description of how learners can vary.

Entry behaviour

The entry behaviour of the learner is a term applied to the prior knowledge and life/professional experiences that the learner brings to each new learning situation. For example, the physiotherapy student entering his or her first clinical placement might exhibit the following entry behaviour:

- aged 20
- A-level background in biology, statistics and psychology
- has successfully completed 1 year of an honours degree course in physiotherapy
- has completed some observation of physiotherapy services prior to taking up the university course.

All these factors may have an effect on how the learner performs in the clinical education setting.

The learner's host institution will supply you with details of what physiotherapy skills/knowledge should have been acquired by the learner prior to commencing the clinical placement, and also what clinical experience the learner has already had. They will not, as a rule, give you specific details of the learner's age and educational abilities and achievements prior to entering the present course. You may find it useful to broaden your knowledge of the learner's entry behaviour when you meet them for the first time. It may give you useful clues as to whether you should modify your approach to facilitation in order to get the best out of each student. You may even wish to adapt your plans to take account of their prior experience in order to avoid repetition.

You might encounter a learner with a completely different entry behaviour:

- a 45-year-old mature student
- work experience as a physiotherapy helper for 4 years prior to entering a physiotherapy degree course
- already holds a degree qualification in biological sciences
- has successfully completed 2 years of the undergraduate programme in physiotherapy
- is now commencing the ninth clinical education placement.

Obviously, the two learners whose entry behaviours have been described will have different needs and abilities. You will need to take this into consideration when planning both local and personal objectives, and also when considering methods of facilitation you might use in the process.

Planning the local objectives

As you have seen in Section 2, core placement objectives for each speciality will already have been set by the host institution, normally in consultation with senior clinicians.

Students will have been given a copy of these core objectives before they enter each new placement so that they can prepare for the new experience. This preparation could include background reading or revision of the appropriate technical skills required. Local objectives (see Section 2 for examples) may also be provided in advance by the clinical educator at each placement setting. These local objectives are written to reflect the experience that the specific placement has to offer, taking account of the constraints that may exist.

ACTIVITY 11.4

Obtain a copy of the core objectives pertaining to your speciality from your host institution. Write some local placement objectives which reflect the experience you can offer the student learner within the constraints you have already identified.

If you have already developed some local placement objectives, review these now and make sure they are still appropriate.

Planning the implementation process

In planning how the placement will be implemented, you need to consider the entry behaviour, the core objectives identified by the host institution, the local objectives you have identified and also the learning environment that will be created for the learning experience (see Section 6 for details of the learning environment). Given the information you have about the learner's stage of education and the spectrum of objectives you have identified that are to be fulfilled by the learner if the placement is to be successfully completed, you must now plan how you can best facilitate this learning process. For example, is an induction period necessary? If so, what does the learner need to know about the department, the staff and the working environment? Does the learner need to read the department's safety regulations or the department's standards document? Does the student need to observe your practice for a short period of time before being given responsibility for their own caseload, however small?

ACTIVITY 11.5

Plan the induction period for a learner who is new to your clinical environment. Outline the activities which must take place, who will be responsible for the induction process, and how long it will take.

It is always useful to remember that, given the opportunity, some learners would be quite content to observe for the whole of their clinical placement! However, this is not the best way to gain hands-on experience, and therefore a balance must be struck between induction and actual clinical practice.

Following induction, the learner moves into a protected clinical practice environment. You, the educator, provide that environment and help to ensure safe practice. But how do you facilitate the taking of responsibility, organisation of caseload skills, problem-solving skills, examination and assessment skills, technical skills and interpersonal skills, and socialisation of the learner from student to health professional, whilst also ensuring that the learner experiences sufficient clinical contact? All these elements need to be addressed in some way. There is no right or wrong way for these things to occur, but it is important always to remember your status as a role model for the learner. Review Section 4 if you need help in planning the implementation process.

ACTIVITY 11.6

Make a day-to-day plan of the learning experience after the induction period. Set times aside for clinical practice and other clinical contact. Timetable meetings between yourself and the learner and state what purpose these meetings will serve. Include any other activities you feel will be needed.

Will you involve other health professionals in this learning experience? If so, how and why? What resources are available to enhance the learner's experience, e.g. ward rounds, observation of surgery, library resources, etc.? What methods of facilitation might you use, e.g. observation, small group teaching, encouraging attendance at in-service lectures?

Be as specific as possible about how the clinical education programme will be arranged, what it will include, who will be involved, and what methods of facilitation will be utilised.

Planning assessment procedures

Normally, host institutions will provide you with an assessment form for each learner, with a set of criteria for marking performance. Often, these forms will have been designed by a combination of academic tutors and clinicians (see Appendix 2 for an example of an assessment form.)

Assessed items often include professionalism, safety, examination and assessment skills, technical skills and interpersonal skills.

A student's performance in these areas is assessed continuously while on placement. The assessment forms vary from one host institution to another, but essentially they assess the same fundamental skills and characteristics.

Most institutions ask that clinical educators make an assessment of learners halfway through the clinical education period, so that the students can obtain feedback on how they are performing. This should enable the students to improve their performance by the end of the placement, and constitutes a modified criterion-referenced assessment (see Section 8). In theory, every student should be capable of achieving 100%, given an unlimited period of time in any placement.

The assessment of clinical practice is very important and, in some universities, marks given by clinical educators are used in the calculation of final degree awards.

The use of the assessment form is therefore not to be taken lightly, and you need to make sure that you are fully informed about its structure, the marking guidelines to be used and criteria for assessment before you begin your clinical educator's role. It is vital that each learner gains accurate feedback on their performance so that they can continue to improve.

ACTIVITY 11.7

Obtain copies of the assessment forms used by each host institution that places students in your workplace. Read them thoroughly, compare them, and make sure you understand the marking system.

Think carefully of ways in which you will assess whether certain criteria have been met – use Section 8 to help you. Review the section on assessment fully and see if you feel the example assessment form given in Appendix 2 fulfils all the criteria of a good assessment.

So far, we have talked about the formal assessment process which is necessary to determine whether or not a student has successfully completed a clinical placement.

ACTIVITY 11.8

Think of ways in which you might informally assess whether learning is taking or has taken place, e.g. question and answer sessions, reviewing X-rays, observing practice.

For each method you list, write a short rationale explaining how the method will be used, what it will assess, and at what stage in the placement it will be used.

Planning the evaluation of the placement

Evaluation occurs as the final part of the cycle, but at this planning stage you need to develop an idea of how you will evaluate the learning experience. You will want to know how the learner felt about all aspects of it.

Most host institutions ask learners to fill out a placement evaluation form. An example is given in Section 9. The form is obviously concerned with the student's perception of the quality of the experience, and this is very dependent upon the nature of the working relationship which has developed between the learner and the clinical educator, as well as upon other factors.

In addition, some educators design evaluation forms for their own personal use. The advantage of this is that the evaluation form is then specific to a particular educator/placement, and in this way educators can seek feedback on factors that are particularly relevant to them. For example, they may want to find out whether or not the learner found them approachable.

ACTIVITY 11.9

Design an evaluation form which could be used to evaluate a learning experience within your workplace. Ask some colleagues to review the form to see if it is understandable.

Now make a list of other ways in which a placement might be evaluated. Refer to the section on evaluation for ideas to add to your list, and suggest when and how this evaluation might be carried out. An example of how evaluation can take place is by committee procedures, i.e. quality groups could be expanded to include student input, and issues pertaining to the quality of a placement could be discussed in open forum.

Having planned the learning experience, you are now ready for the learner to arrive, so the next stage in the cycle commences. Review Sections 4 and 7 now; they will help you with the design of the learning experience.

Designing the learning

This is the stage during which the planned learning experience is tailored to the needs of the individual student. As part of a new learner's induction programme, it is normal practice for an educator to spend some time discussing learning needs.

In conjunction with the learner, the educator will identify the learner's needs in terms of interpersonal and psycho-motor skills development and in terms of what knowledge needs to be acquired and how it can be used. Section 8, which was on assessment, introduced 'Bloom's Taxonomy of Learning'. This is often a useful tool for the clinical educator when trying to find the level at which the learner's abilities lie, in terms of knowledge, attitudes and skills acquisition; i.e. the learner may have acquired factual information relevant to the placement, but can they yet use this information to make clear decisions? For learners on their first placement, this is usually not the case, but more experienced learners may well be able to synthesise information early on in a placement and have well-developed clinical reasoning skills.

ACTIVITY 11.10

Revisit Bloom's taxonomies in Section 8 so that you are familiar with the hierarchies of learning.

Having identified an individual learner's needs, personal objectives can now be set. These are often based on the local placement objectives, but will be more specific and will include objectives relating to some of the gaps identified in the learner's knowledge which it is felt can be filled in this placement. The importance of this setting of personal objectives was highlighted in Section 7.

Some educators prefer to use a learning contract (re-read the subsection on learning contracts in Section 7 by way of review).

Also at this stage, the learning experience plan can be firmly mapped out or modified in order to fulfil more specifically the personal objectives of the learner concerned. Much will depend on factors such as the learner's style of learning, prior experiences, maturity and motivation, etc. (see Section 5 on factors influencing learning for further detail).

Once the individual learning needs have been identified, you should now consider what scope exists to facilitate learning in the desired areas. Also bear in mind your local constraints. For example, the learner may have identified a need to gain more experience of postoperative care following knee surgery, but it may be the case that there are few patients of this nature referred to your unit for treatment. This is a constraint that cannot necessarily be overcome.

As a result of your first meeting with the learner, you may now begin to think of more appropriate methods of facilitating the learning and you may want to alter the sequence of the learning programme in some way to account for gaps in the student's knowledge/abilities. For example, the learner may need more experience in examination and assessment of simple conditions before taking on more complex challenges.

You may decide that certain resources are now superfluous, while others may seem more essential; for example, there may be a need to use more X-rays in teaching than was previously anticipated. You may also feel that more frequent meetings for discussion are required than you had previously timetabled.

Implementing the learning experience

Having thoroughly planned the learning experience in the last two stages, both you and the learner now have objectives which are clearly identified. The actual implementation of the experience should be reasonably straightforward, but throughout this stage you must remember the elements of your role that were examined in Section 2. The need to be continuously assessing performance and giving constructive and meaningful feedback in order for the student to be given the opportunity to improve must not be underestimated. This means carefully deciding how, when and where you will assess the learner's knowledge, psycho-motor skills, technical abilities and interpersonal skills, and also their ability to demonstrate the integration of these skills while keeping their patient at their ease (review Section 7 in order to remind yourself of the value of feedback).

Think of when and how you will give the learner feedback. It may also be necessary at some point (or points) in the placement to review the original personal objectives, as some may have become redundant in the case of a gifted and highly motivated learner (in other words, some of them may already have been fulfilled); for others, the objectives set may have been too high for their abilities, and there may therefore be a need to modify them to make them more achievable.

Finally, throughout the implementation process you should be aware of all the factors that may influence learning. Review Section 5 for further details.

Assessing learning

Assessment planning was dealt with earlier on in this section, but it is worth noting again that performance is most commonly assessed on a continuous basis, with the student given formal feedback halfway through the placement period; another formal assessment then takes place at the end of the placement. Obviously, feedback on performance occurs frequently on an informal basis during the rest of the period – following observation periods, discussion periods and question periods, etc. – and this feedback usually occurs on a one-to-one basis.

Once an assessment has been carried out, its results should be analysed. Where are the weak areas? What can be done to help? What must be done in order to improve performance? Often the assessment is discussed with the learner and forms the basis of a final, frank feedback session. Sometimes learners are encouraged to assess their own performance in tandem with the educator, and then an assessment of performance is agreed jointly.

Never be afraid to tell a learner the truth. If a learner's performance is poor, they must be told as soon as is practically possible, so that time and the opportunity to improve is not lost. Equally, the student who demonstrates an excellent performance should know that their performance has been of a high standard in order to feel satisfaction and confidence in their abilities.

Evaluating the learning experience

This is one of the later stages in the cycle. Normally, as was noted earlier in this section, a standard evaluation form is used which is often provided by the host institution. Evaluation is useful for the host institution, for the student and for the educator. Don't be afraid to evaluate a learning experience for yourself, using any method you feel comfortable with. The host institution will supply their own evaluation forms so that they can monitor the standard of each of the clinical placements they use. If you choose to evaluate for yourself, you may well keep your own results to yourself, or you may wish to share them with one or two colleagues or with your line manager.

Results from the university's student evaluation forms are sometimes fed back to clinical educators individually, but within the host institution they are fed back through the university's quality assurance system, and action is taken if necessary to withdraw students from placements which appear to be consistently unsatisfactory. See Section 9 for details of the importance and uses of evaluation.

Feedback

Feedback can be given on various factors: a student's performance during the placement; the educator's perception of success or otherwise during the placement; the assessment; and the evaluation of placement. Feedback may be given to learners, clinical educators or visiting tutors from the various host institutions. Clinical educators will often have the ability to feed information directly into host institutions by way of attendance at course boards or boards of study and/or by input into course development teams. Obviously, the issue of feedback is much wider than just the individual's perspective; feedback can be made to one's profession, to a management hierarchy, or perhaps to an audit committee.

Finally, during the design of any learning experience, the educator must be aware of the need to reflect on the learning experience, taking into account the results of any evaluation that has taken place and, where necessary, implementing changes to improve the quality of the learning experience. Do changes need to be made to any of the stages of the cycle? If so, these changes need to be taken into consideration when planning further placements.

Look at the curriculum cycle in detail again, and see how the various stages may be dependent upon other stages; for example, feedback on learning could affect planning, design, implementation and evaluation.

ACTIVITY 11.11

Using the curriculum model provided, design a 4-week placement within your own speciality for a student who is nearing completion of their clinical education programme and the end of their degree course. Also highlight how the design could be made suitable for a novice learner.

ACTIVITY 11.12

This activity, because of its practical nature and the real-life scenario, is likely to take in excess of 5-6 weeks.

Having planned a hypothetical education placement, you now need to see how the model works in practice.

If you are due to take on an educator's role, carry out the same process you carried out in the previous activities for this new learning situation. This time, however, you will be in the position of being able to assess, evaluate, give feedback, and reflect on the process, as well as taking part in the actual implementation of the programme.

If you are not in a position to plan a clinical placement curriculum personally, then find a clinical educator in your environment who is, and try to plan a placement together.

During the whole process, make detailed notes. First, make notes of the planning stages and then make notes containing your reflections on the events as they take place, e.g. changing constraints and action plans to overcome these constraints, taking into account caseload changes, student problems, etc.

Make a record of learning contracts and objectives which are set, particularly those set in liaison with the student. Analyse the feedback obtained from the learner or the learner's visiting tutor, together with the results of any assessments carried out, whether formative or summative. Finally, reflect on the whole process, exploring avenues for feedback or improvement. Where appropriate, return to your planning model to see if changes need to be made to any stage in the design. Make a note of these changes, explaining why they are necessary and how they will be implemented.

As you can see, you have just completed some research into your own activities as a clinical educator. Research, however, is only useful if the findings are shared. Think now about how you will share this information; for example, you may wish to present an overview of the learning experience to other physiotherapists in your workplace. You may, on the other hand, wish to write up the process for publication in a journal, or you may wish to discuss your plans and findings with a visiting tutor from the host institution.

Summary

Having completed this section, you should now feel more confident in your role as a clinical educator, in both global and specific senses. You may feel that you wish to contribute actively to the future developments which will inevitably occur in the clinical education forum in light of the issues raised in Section 10. In order for you to enhance your role, Section 12 includes further information which will be of interest to those who wish to improve their skills further and to gain more formal recognition for their experience in clinical education.

REFERENCE
Rowntree D 1982 Educational technology in curriculum development, 2nd edn. Harper & Row, London, p 21

12 Further information

Opportunities for further study

For details of courses in education and other relevant postgraduate courses, see the Chartered Society of Physiotherapy's (1995) Postgraduate Study Pack available from the Education Department at the Chartered Society of Physiotherapy, 14 Bedford Row, London, WC1R 4ED (price £5).

A Physiotherapy Access to Continuing Education (PACE) catalogue containing all the courses recognised by the Chartered Society of Physiotherapy is available from the Chartered Society of Physiotherapy, 14 Bedford Row, London, WC1R 4ED (price £3.50 per copy). This catalogue is updated quarterly.

Bibliography

Professional issues

Barclay J 1994 In good hands. Butterworth Heinemann, Oxford

Chartered Society of Physiotherapy 1991 Standards for clinical education. Chartered Society of Physiotherapy, London

Chartered Society of Physiotherapy 1991 Curriculum of study. Chartered Society of Physiotherapy, London

Chartered Society of Physiotherapy 1992 Professional development diary. Chartered Society of Physiotherapy, London

Chartered Society of Physiotherapy 1994 Centenary Issue, Physiotherapy Journal. Chartered Society of Physiotherapy, London

Chartered Society of Physiotherapy 1994 Guidelines for good practice for the education of clinical educators. Chartered Society of Physiotherapy, London

Chartered Society of Physiotherapy 1994 PACE information paper. Chartered Society of Physiotherapy, London

Jones R 1991 Management in physiotherapy. Radcliffe Medical Press, Oxford

Wicksteed J 1948 The growth of the profession. Edward Arnold and Company, London

Managing and facilitating learning

Abercrombie M L 1993 The human nature of learning: selections from the work of M L Abercrombie. OU Press/SRHE, Milton Keynes

Boud D 1981 Developing autonomy in learning. Kogan Page, London

Boud D, Keogh R, Wallter D (eds) 1985 Reflection: turning experience into learning. Kogan Page, London

Brandes D, Ginnis P 1986 A guide to student centred learning. Blackwell, Oxford

Brown G 1988 Effective teaching in higher education. Methuen, London

Brown S, Knight P 1994 Assessing learning in higher education. Kogan Page, London

Buzan T 1974 Use your head. BBC Publications, Rugby

Collier G 1982 Resource based learning in higher and continuing education. Croom Helm, Beckenham

Connel R W 1987 Gender and power. Allen Unwin, London

Cotterell A, Ennals R (with Briggs J H) 1988 Advanced information technology in education and training. Edward Arnold, London

Cross V 1992 Using learning contracts in clinical education. A handbook for students and clinical educators (available from V.Cross, Queen Elizabeth School of Physiotherapy, Queen Elizabeth Medical Centre, Edgbaston, Birmingham, BI5 2SH)

Dennison B, Kirk R 1990 Do, review, learn, apply: a simple guide to experimental learning. Blackwell Education, London

Entwistle N 1988 Styles of learning and teaching. David Fullerton Publishers, London

Eraunt M 1994 Developing professional knowledge and competence. Falmer Press, London

Good T, Brophy J 1990 Educational psychology. Longman, New York

Hammond M, Collins R 1991 Self directed learning: critical practice. Kogan Page, London

Hodgeson V E, Mann S J, Snell R (eds) 1987 Beyond distance teaching towards open learning. Society for Research into Higher Education and Open University Press, Milton Keynes

Holmberg B 1985 Status and trends of distance learning. Lector Publishing, Lund Sweden

Illich I 1977 Disabling professions. Marion Boyers, New York

Jacques D 1991 Learning in groups. Kogan Page, London

Jessop G 1991 Outcomes: NVQs and the emerging models of education and learning. Falmer Press, London

Knowles M 1990 The adult learner: a neglected species, 4th edn. Gulf Publishing, Houston

Kolb D A 1984 Experiential Learning: experience as a source of learning and development. Prentice Hall, New Jersey

Marton F, Hounsell D, Entwistle N 1995 (eds) The experience of learning, 2nd edn. Scottish Academic Press, Edinburgh

McGill I, Beaty E 1995 Effective action learning: a guide for professionals, managers and educational developers. Kogan Page, London.

Nisbet J D, Schucksmith 1986 Learning strategies. Routledge, London

Ramsden P 1992 Learning to teach in higher education. Routledge, London

Rogers C 1983 Freedom to learn. Charles E Merrill, Ohio

Rogers J 1977 Adults learning. Open University Press, Milton Keynes

Rowntree D 1989 Assessing students. How shall we know them? Kogan Page, London

Schon D A 1987 Educating the reflective practitioner. Jossey Bass, San Francisco

Warner S, McGill I (eds) 1989 Making sense of experimental learning. Society for Research in Higher Education and Open University Press. Milton Keynes

Role development

American Physical Therapy Association 1992 (eds) Clinical education: an anthology. American Physical Therapy Association, Baltimore

Argris C, Schon D 1974 Theory into practice: increasing professional effectiveness. Jossey Bass, San Francisco

Benner P 1984 From novice to expert: excellence and power in critical nursing practice. Addision Wesley, California

Boud D, Keogh R, Wallter D (eds) 1985 Reflection: turning experience into learning. Kogan Page, London

Cohen L, Manion L 1989 Research methods in education. Routledge, London

Eraut M 1994 Developing professional knowledge and competence. Falmer Press, London

French S, Neville S, Laing J 1994 Teaching and learning: a guide for therapists. Butterworth Heinemann, Oxford

Hicks C M 1995 Research for physiotherapists, 2nd edn. Churchill Livingstone, Edinburgh

Patton M Q 1990 Qualitative evaluation and research methods, 2nd edn. Sage, Newbury Park, CA

Schon D A 1987 Educating the reflective practitioner. Jossey Bass, San Francisco

Stewart C 1988 Effective speaking. Pan, London

Yaxley B G 1991 Developing teachers' theories of teaching – a touchstone approach. Falmer Press, London

Yelloly M, Henkel M 1995 Learning and teaching in social work. Jessica Kingsley, London

Curriculum studies for health professionals

Bound D, Feletti G (eds) 1991 The challenge of problem based learning. Kogan Page, London

Burrell T W 1988 Curriculum design and development. Prentice Hall, Hemel Hempstead

Fullan M G 1991 The new meaning of educational change. Cassell, London

Golby M et al 1982 Curriculum design. Croom Helm, London

Guba E G, Lincoln Y S 1987 Effective evaluation. Jossey Bass, San Francisco

Jessup G 1991 Outcomes, NVQs and the emerging model of education and training. Falmer Press, London

Lawton D 1983 Curriculum studies and educational planning. Hodder & Stoughton, London

Murphy R, Torrance H (eds) 1987 Evaluating education: issues and method. Harper & Row, London

Pendleton S and Myles A (eds) 1991 Curriculum planning in nursing education. Edward Arnold, London

Skilbeck M 1984 School based curriculum development. Harper & Row, London

Stenhouse L 1975 An introduction to curriculum research and development. Heinemann, London

Taylor P, Richards C 1985 An introduction to curriculum studies. NFER-Nelson, Berkshire

Appendix 1—Factors which influence learning as identified by learners

Negative factors

Disparity in levels of marking between placements
Written feedback not matching verbal feedback
Having been expected to have an enquiring attitude in the School, I was sometimes made to feel that questions in the clinical situation were unwelcome and that I was being insubordinate for asking them
Found it difficult to cope with change in supervisors approach and attitude from one clinical placement to another. Their expectations can vary enormously and I am supposed to know what they want from me
Supervisors being away for part of the time
Half-way reports not given, or not given on time
Staff seeming too busy
Lack of preparation on arrival/disorganised
Being the only student at a hospital
Being watched a lot
Lack of 'hands-on' in some placements
Being criticised in front of patients/other staff
Extra work set that clashes with course work

Accommodation

Prowlers, poor security, feeling unsafe
Not clean/smelly
Noisy, can't work
Telephones stolen
No heating – difficult to dry towels after hydrotherapy sessions.
Cockroaches in bedrooms ('but I now know how to kill cockroaches without spreading their eggs')
No desks in rooms
Kitchen facilities inadequate, no hot water
By myself in the accommodation

No library facilities at the hospital
Library closes too early

Positive factors

Physiotherapists helpful and welcoming
Felt a very welcome department/very friendly
Feeling like part of the team
Tutorials/teaching sessions very useful
'Senior staff making sure you are OK in the accommodation – bring you extra blankets!'

Appreciated not being treated as an extra basic grade, but as students and therefore a manageable work load

Help with research project

Relaxed manner of supervision

Friendly staff – invited us to social events

Inservice training very useful

Help available when needed

Feeling like one of the staff

Good balance of teaching and observing

My Senior was very approachable

Opportunity to watch sometimes

Busy but not over stretched

Practising on the clinician

Wide range of conditions treated

Sticking to the students 30 hours/week

Books and articles available

Good library facilities appreciated when available

Nice to have a room with a desk

Contact with students from another School

Carrot cake from cake shop at Guy's

Canteen food, when good, is *always* mentioned

Appendix 2 – Example clinical placement assessment form

Please fill in this form with reference to the criteria listed in the clinicians' document.

Name of student _____

Placement: Service _____ Unit _____

Date of work: from _____ to _____

The contents of this form are confidential.

Area of assessment	Comments	Grade
1. Professionalism		
2. Knowledge and understanding		
3. Examination and assessment of patients		
4. Treatment of patients		

Area of assessment	Comment	Grade
5. Evaluation of treatment		
6. Skills		
7. Communication		
8. Reaction to advice		
9. Initiative/adaptability		
10. Reliability		
11. Responsibility		
Area of assessment	Comment	Grade

Mid-placement assessment

The section below should be completed half way through placement

(Please grade as satisfactory or unsatisfactory by reference to lists of criteria in clinical educators' document).

Grade ☐   (S = satisfactory   U = unsatisfactory)

If the student is NOT satisfactory at this stage please complete the following section stating what advice the student has received to assist in improving their performance on this placement.

Signatures:-   Clinical educator _____ Date _____
                      Student _____ Date _____

Final assessment
(The section below should be completed at the end of the placement)

General comments, including those from other departmental staff, at end of placement.

Comments from visiting lecturer.

Date(s) absent:-

Signatures:-   Clinical educator _____

University staff _____

Student _____

N.B. The student should NOT sign the report until they have discussed its contents with their clinical educator (clinician).

In working out a percentage for the *final* assessment of the placement the following table should be used.

Guidelines for marking

6/ All criteria consistently maintained at a very high level
5/ Majority of criteria consistently at a high level, remainder acceptable
4/ Some criteria at a high level, remainder acceptable
3/ All criteria consistently at an acceptable level
2/ Majority of criteria at an acceptable level, some weakness that should improve with experience
1/ Majority of criteria at an unacceptable level with minimum at an acceptable level
0/ No criteria at an acceptable level

Section	Mark	Multiplied by	TOTAL
1. Professionalism		1	
2. Knowledge		3	
3. Assessment of patients		3	
4. Treatment of patients		3	
5. Evaluation of treatment		3	
6. Skills		3	
7. Communication		3	
8. Reaction to advice		1	
9. Initiative/adaptability		1	
10. Reliability		1	
11. Responsibility		1	

SAFETY (This section must be passed).
Is the student generally safe in this area of clinical practice?   YES/NO
(Please refer to criteria).

Total for the Placement (formula) $= \dfrac{100 \times total}{138}$

Percentage for the placement

Suggested criteria for specified areas of assessment of the clinical report form in placements 1–4

1. **Professionalism**
   a) Appearance
   - Should appear neat, tidy, well groomed and clean.
   - Should wear appropriate attire for differing work situations.

   b) Punctuality
   - Should arrive punctually in time for work.
   - Should demonstrate prompt time keeping with patients.
   - Should demonstrate punctuality with regard to arrangements made with staff.

   c) Rapport with patients
   - Should demonstrate consideration and understanding with regard to patients.

   d) Rapport with colleagues
   - Should demonstrate consideration and understanding with regard to colleagues.

2. **Knowledge**
   - Should demonstrate a good basic knowledge of the common conditions likely to be met on the placement and those conditions encountered during the placement. May require some assistance in seeking further information.

3. **Examination and assessment of patients**
   - demonstrate the ability to extract relevant information from patients and the patients' notes, but may require some guidance particularly with more extensive notes.
   - Should demonstrate the ability to select and use appropriate clinical tests for the condition being assessed, but at this stage may require some guidance in the selection and assistance in the performance of tests.
   - Should demonstrate some ability to interpret the results of the assessment procedures correctly.

4. **Treatment of patients**
   a) Appropriate selection
   - Should demonstrate the appropriate selection of treatment techniques from the knowledge gained from assessment of the patient but will require some guidance.

   b) Use of practical skills
   - Should demonstrate the appropriate use of practical skills related to the need of the patient being treated but may need assistance with new or more complicated techniques.

   c) Patient care
   - Should demonstrate patient care but may need some advice to become more effective.

5. **Evaluation of treatment**
   a) Effectiveness
   - Should be able to assess the effectiveness of treatment but needing some guidance.

   b) Progression
   - Should be able to suggest appropriate progression or modification of treatment plans but may need guidance at this stage.

6. Skills
- Should perform practical skills efficiently and show some ability to apply and progress.
- Should perform practical skills autonomously at most times.
- Should demonstrate appropriate modifications with confidence in most areas.
- Should be receptive to the introduction of new skills.

7. Communication
  a) Notes
  - Should keep neat, comprehensive accurate notes using POMR or another acceptable convention but may require advice to improve note-taking techniques and modifications appropriate to the placement.

  b) Letters
  - Should demonstrate the ability to write relevant letters or reports to other members of the interdisciplinary team but requiring assistance at times.

  c) Verbal with colleagues
  - Should demonstrate effective verbal communication with colleagues but may require some assistance.

  d) Verbal with patients
  - Should demonstrate effective verbal communication with patients.

8. Reaction to advice
- Should be receptive to advice.
- Should be able to accept valid and constructive criticism.
- Should be able to act according to advice given.

9. Initiative/adaptability
- Should manage time effectively but may require some advice.
- Should show initiative in planning their case load but may require some advice to improve planning techniques.
- Should show a level of initiative commensurate with the stage of professional development – may require guidance.
- Should demonstrate the ability to adapt to variations in conditions regarding patients or treatment facilities but at this stage may require guidance and/or assistance.

10. Reliability
- Should be dependable in implementing agreed arrangements and procedures.
- Should demonstrate an acceptable level of self organisation but may require advice.
- Should be trusted to work alone where appropriate.

11. Responsibility
- Should demonstrate a keen sense of responsibility towards patients.
- Should be prepared for personal inconvenience if the situation demands.
- Should demonstrate a level of responsibility

commensurate with their stage of education – will still require fairly close supervision particularly when first introduced to the placement.

SAFETY
- Should observe general safety precautions at all times.
- Should demonstrate safe patient handling.
- Should demonstrate safe use of equipment.

Suggested criteria for specified areas of assessment of the clinical report form in placements 5–8

I. Professionalism

a) Appearance
- Should appear neat, tidy, well groomed and clean.
- Should wear appropriate attire for differing work situations.

b) Punctuality
- Should arrive punctually in time for work.
- Should demonstrate prompt time keeping with patients.
- Should demonstrate punctuality with regard to arrangements made with staff.

c) Rapport with patients
- Should demonstrate consideration and understanding with regard to patients.

d) Rapport with colleagues
- Should demonstrate consideration and understanding with regard to colleagues.

2. Knowledge
- Should demonstrate a good basic knowledge of the common conditions likely to be met on the placement and those conditions encountered during the placement
- this should be approaching the standard expected of a newly qualified physiotherapist. Where a condition is unusual the student should demonstrate the ability to discover information for himself/herself.

3. Examination and assessment of patient
- demonstrate the ability to extract relevant information from patients and the patients' notes with assistance only in complex cases.
- Should demonstrate the ability to select and use appropriate clinical tests for the condition being assessed and where techniques are new the initiative to discover the appropriate tests for themselves.
- Should demonstrate the ability to interpret the results of the assessment procedures correctly.

4. Treatment of patients

a) Appropriate selection
- Should demonstrate the appropriate selection of treatment techniques from the knowledge gained from assessment of the patient requiring guidance only in complex cases.

b) Use of practical skills
- Should demonstrate the appropriate use of practical skills related to the needs of the patient

being treated with suitable modifications where appropriate.

c) Patient care — Should demonstrate patient care.

5. Evaluation of treatment

a) Effectiveness — Should be able to make a realistic assessment of the effectiveness of their treatment.

b) Progression — Should be able to suggest appropriate progression or modification of treatment plans.

6. Skills

- Should perform practical skills efficiently and show well developed ability to apply and progress their application.
- Should perform practical skills autonomously.
- Should demonstrate appropriate modifications with confidence.
- Should be receptive to the introduction of new skills.

7. Communication

a) Notes — Should keep neat, comprehensive accurate notes using POMR or another acceptable convention.

b) Letters — Should demonstrate the ability to write relevant letters or reports to other members of the interdisciplinary team.

c) Verbal with colleagues — Should demonstrate confident and effective verbal communication with colleagues.

d) Verbal with patients — Should demonstrate effective verbal communication with patients with confidence.

8. Reaction to advice

- Should be receptive to advice and seek advice when appropriate.
- Should be able to accept valid and constructive criticism and show a willingness to seek criticism in the search for self improvement.
- Should be able to act according to advice given.

9. Initiative/adaptability

- Should manage time effectively.
- Should show initiative in planning their case load.
- Should show a level of initiative commensurate with the stage of professional development but recognising when it is appropriate to seek advice.
- Should demonstrate the ability to adapt to variations in conditions regarding patients or treatment facilities.

10. Reliability

- Should be dependable in implementing agreed arrangements and procedures.
- Should demonstrate an acceptable level of self organisation adapting quickly to the demands of a new environment.
- Should be trusted to work alone where appropriate.

11. Responsibility

- Should demonstrate a keen sense of responsibility towards patients.
- Should be prepared for personal inconvenience if the situation demands.

– Should demonstrate a level of responsibility commensurate with their stage of education.

SAFETY

– Should observe general safety precautions at all times.
– Should demonstrate safe patient handling.
– Should demonstrate safe use of equipment.

Appendix 3 – Example clinical placement evaluation form

Clinical Centre:
Hospital/Unit:
Clinical Speciality:
Placement Dates:
Student Year:
PMA Result:
Name of Clinical Educator:
Name of College Link Tutor:

1) **ORIENTATION/INTEGRATION**

Please tick the appropriate box:

How comprehensive and helpful was the induction material?

Very good ☐   Good ☐   Average ☐   Barely adequate ☐   Unhelpful ☐

Any comments:

How well integrated were you into the team?

| Fully integrated ☐ | Well integrated ☐ | Reasonably well integrated ☐ | Poorly integrated ☐ | Not integrated at all ☐ |

Any comments:

Please comment on:

a) Attendance at in-service education.

b) Opportunities to meet the other members of the multidisciplinary team.

c) Library facilities.

State if these were not available to you.

2) CLINICAL EXPERIENCE

a) <u>College Preparation</u>

How well did College-based studies prepare you for the theoretical requirements of the placement?

Very well ☐   Well ☐   Adequately ☐   Inadequately ☐   Not at all ☐

Comments:

How well did College-based studies prepare you for the practical requirements of the placement?

Very well ☐   Well ☐   Adequately ☐   Inadequately ☐   Not at all ☐

Comments:

b) <u>Patient/Client Selection</u>

I saw an appropriate selection of patients/clients.

Strongly agree ☐   Agree ☐   Disagree ☐   Strongly disagree ☐

My patients/clients load was appropriate.

Strongly agree ☐   Agree ☐   Disagree ☐   Strongly disagree ☐

Please make any supporting comments you think helpful: -

c) <u>Objectives</u>

I was able to achieve the core objectives of the placement.

Strongly agree ☐   Agree ☐   Disagree ☐   Strongly disagree ☐

Comments/explanation:

I negotiated and set local and personal objectives.

Strongly agree ☐   Agree ☐   Disagree ☐   Strongly disagree ☐

Please make any supporting comments you think helpful.

I was able to achieve the local and personal objectives.

Strongly agree ☐   Agree ☐   Disagree ☐   Strongly disagree ☐

d) <u>Supervision and Teaching</u>

The clinical educator encouraged the development of skills relevant to the placement.

Strongly agree ☐   Agree ☐   Disagree ☐   Strongly disagree ☐

Any comments:

I had regular and appropriate access to my clinical educator.

Strongly agree ☐   Agree ☐   Disagree ☐   Strongly disagree ☐

Any comments:

The clinical educator provided positive feedback and constructive criticism when appropriate.

Strongly agree ☐   Agree ☐   Disagree ☐   Strongly disagree ☐

Any comments:

Please make any supporting comments you think helpful.

3) TRAVEL & ACCOMMODATION

Please comment under this section if applicable.

4) GENERAL COMMENTS

Please make any general comments that you have not had the opportunity to make:-

Thank you for your help in the completion of this evaluation form.

Figure 9.4 Example of a clinical evaluation form

Glossary

Terms relating to clinical education

clinical education – the essential and extensive element of healthcare professional courses which provides the focus for integration of academic and practice-based learning in a work–based setting

clinical education partnership – the working relationship between clinical educator, learner, college-based educator and clinical manager, that is essential for successful planning, organisation and conduct of the placement experience

clinical educator – an experienced work–based professional practitioner who accepts responsibility for a specific component of the clinical education programme and process.

college link tutor – a member of the university staff who has responsibility for linking with the physiotherapy service and clinical educator and the learner, before, during and after the placement

learner (in the context of this package) – an undergraduate or qualified member of a healthcare profession, who is undertaking a clinically-based education programme

clinical placements – an opportunity for the learner to undertake supervised learning and practice in a relevant setting, where the clinical educator is involved in facilitating learning and assessing professional development

work/practice-based learning – structured opportunities for participants to develop their learning, either within a clinical placement or their own work place

Terms relating to general education

pre-registration education – any three or four year programme of study that leads to the granting of a licence to practice a particular profession and state registration as a member of that profession

post-registration education – any programme of study undertaken following initial professional education and state registration

undergraduate education – any three or four year course programme leading to the award of a first degree

post-graduate education – any programme of study that advances learning beyond undergraduate level

continuing education – any educational activity undertaken following completion of an initial course programme

continuing professional development – ongoing learning by which individuals maintain, enhance and broaden their professional knowledge, understanding and skills

Terms used by college-based educators, universities and professional bodies which relate to health care professional courses and curricula

clinical information days – activities organised by the university which hosts the course, during which college-based educators provide clinical educators with information about the curriculum and assessment programme and requirements

validation – a process during which academic and professional bodies gather information in order to determine whether a course is 'sound', 'sufficient' and delivered with proper formalities

accreditation – the formal recognition of a course

educational philosophy – the educational ethos of a course that shapes its aims and learning outcomes and design

ethos – a set of attitudes and beliefs

integration – to make up as a whole; to make entire

aims – the educational purpose of a course that expresses in general terms the new knowledge, skills, qualities and attitudes that participants should gain

objectives – detailed specification of learning outcomes

taxonomy – classification

teaching methods – the procedures used to deliver a course and to develop participants' learning

assessment – the means by which participants' fulfilment of the aims and learning outcomes of a course is tested

formative – an assessment or evaluation activity that provides feedback during the course of an educational event

summative – an assessment or evaluation, conducted at the end of an educational event that provides information as to its success

criterion – principle or standard by which something is judged

criterion-referenced – performance compared against standard criterion

norm-referenced – performance compared with the norm

evaluation – an activity whereby educators endeavour to find out how successful a educational event has been in realising educational aims, enabling learners to achieve their objectives, planning, providing and facilitating learning

illuminative evaluation – an evaluation strategy which utilises different methods to 'throw light' on a particular problem or issue

ethnographic study – the study of individuals in their social settings

validity – the extent to which an instrument measures what it purports to measure

reliability – the consistency or repeatability of a measure

quality assurance – a positive (based on valid and reliable evidence) declaration of the degree of excellence of something

Terms relating to the teaching and learning process

learning styles – approaches to learning which reflect the individuality of the learner

learning strategies – planned approaches to learning assignments which should be both suitable and task specific

learning process – the entire learning experience created within a course by its educational philosophy and rationale, aims and learning outcomes, structure, teaching and learning methods and assessment procedures

learning outcome – the specific learning that participants should achieve through their completion of the course

self-directed learning (independent learning) – process by which students take responsibility for their own learning, while retaining access to advice and support from tutors

experiential learning – learning gained through professional practice, rather than through the completion of a formal course

analysis – resolution into simpler elements

synthesis – building up, putting together, making a whole out of parts

motivation – excited to action by particular considerations or emotions

intrinsic motivation – a source of motivation which comes from 'within' the individual

extrinsic motivation – a source of motivation that is 'imposed' or 'created' by other people or sets of circumstances

learning experience – participation in any teacher or learner led, academic discipline-orientated or clinically-orientated learning opportunity, in either the college-base or clinical setting

learning environment (milieu) – a setting where educational opportunities are provided and maximized

facilitation – to make easier, to promote

reinforcement – (in an educational context) to support learning though offering opportunities to repeat and consolidate a specific learning experience, or achieve a similar learning outcome by a different means

feedback – useful information or guidelines for future development

learning contract – the formalisation of a negotiated programme of learning for an individual student

constructive criticism – to alert a learner to the need to improve a specific aspect of their performance in a way that does not undermine confidence and draws on the learner's strengths. This includes discussion and identification of strategies to achieve new objectives

reflective practice – a process of reviewing an episode of practice to describe, analyse, evaluate and inform learning about practice. In this way, new learning modifies previous perceptions and understanding, and the application of learning to clinical practice influences treatment approaches and outcomes

Terms associated with contemporary practice issues

multidisciplinary practice – a process whereby various members of the health care team contribute their specific professional expertise to the identification, analysis and management of clients' problems. Their individual contributions are then co-ordinated as a needs related programme of intervention

provider service – a component part of the health service, be it in a unit or department, which offers a service, in the context of this package, to either patients or for clinical placements

market economy – an economy in which the greater part of the activities of production, distribution and exchange are conducted by individual organisations rather than by the government, and in which the government's intervention is kept to a minimum

market forces – the forces of influence which are generated by, and drive a market economy

professional body – the organisation established to, and with the purpose of managing the activities of a profession

professional competence – the ability and capability to demonstrate sufficient and suitable knowledge and skill for the purpose of being included as a member of the specified profession

PACE – physiotherapy access to continuing education

General Whitley Council – one of the councils forming the system of the national negotiating machinery, consisting of employers and unions at the local level of the NHS

portfolio – a collection of documented evidence on a specific subject

professional development diary – a 'diary' in which appropriate evidence of an individual's professional development is recorded, collated and stored

NHSE letters – letters of information, policy or direction, from the National Health Service Executive to healthcare purchasers and providers on specific subjects. A means of communication between the centre and the field